The Game's Trivia....
James Bond *Trivia*

Chad Brenden

Compiled by
Sally Brenden

Trivia Questions by Chad Brenden
Compiled by Sally Brenden

TABLE OF CONTENTS

Dedication

Introduction

Movies Upon Which Questions Are Based

James Bond Actors....................1

Bond Girls....................4

Which James Bond Movie....................7

Actors....................17

The Ladies....................20

Names....................24

Gadgets....................32

Music....................35

Villains....................38

Unpleasant Demises....................43

Missions & Plots....................45

Food & Drink....................47

Locations....................49

Transportation....................51

Weapons a.k.a. Instruments of Death....................53

Signs & Passwords & What Did it Say?....................55

Dates....................58

Numbers....................60

Directors/Producers/Screenwriters....................62

Which Non-James Bond Movie....................64

Miscellaneous Trivia....................69

"Quotes"....................74

I dedicate this to Ian Fleming, Sean Connery, Roger Moore, Peter Sellers, David Niven, Pierce Brosnan, Daniel Craig, and Desmond Llewelyn the 8 men I admire most

and

to my Ma whom I teamed up with in this piece of writing material

and

to the Lord whom is also someone I admire most.

INTRODUCTION

What first brought me to the James Bond series was back in 1998 at the age of 11 I got very easily hooked on the Nintendo 64 James Bond video game “GoldenEye” where my older brother got me into that video game and playing that game is one of the greatest memories of my childhood and then a few years later I started watching the James Bond movies in summer 2002 I started at the age of 15 watching the James Bond series, and the Star Wars series, and the Mission: Impossible movies and at the age of 31 I’m still a fan today.

In November 2007 before Thanksgiving my Mama asked me to try to write James Bond trivia to stump the relatives, and I was exhilarated with the idea and so I tested some of my relatives with James Bond trivia and that’s what started the whole thing after all James Bond and Veggie Tales are two things I grew up with.

I also wrote like 969 James Bond trivia index cards and most of them have a different question on both sides so I actually wrote thousands of James Bond trivia questions.

MOVIES UPON WHICH QUESTIONS ARE BASED

- Casino Royale (1954 TV version)
  This is the first on-screen adaptation of Ian Fleming's James Bond character. It was featured on television as an episode of the dramatic anthology series Climax!, hosted by William Lundigan, airing on CBS from 1954 to 1958. While it may be considered an "unofficial" James Bond movie by many, Chad has included this in his trivia questions.
- Dr. No (1962)
- From Russia with Love (1963)
- Goldfinger (1964)
- Thunderball (1965)
- Casino Royale (1967)
  This is also called the comedy version of Casino Royale
- You Only Live Twice (1967)
- On Her Majesty's Secret Service (1969)
- Diamonds Are Forever (1971)
- Live and Let Die (1973)
- The Man with the Golden Gun (1974)
- The Spy Who Loved Me (1977)
- Moonraker (1979)
- For Your Eyes Only (1981)
- Octopussy (1983)
- Never Say Never Again (1983)
- A View to a Kill (1985)
- The Living Daylights (1987)
- Licence to Kill (1989)
- GoldenEye (1995)
- Tomorrow Never Dies (1997)
- The World Is Not Enough (1999)
- Die Another Day (2002)
- Casino Royale (2006)
- Quantum of Solace (2008)
- Skyfall (2012)
- SPECTRE (2015)

JAMES BOND ACTORS

1. So far how many actors played James Bond?
   (Per list of Movies Upon Which Questions Are Based)
   10

2. Who are the 10 actors who have played James Bond?
   (Per list Movies Upon Which questions Are Based)
   Barry Nelson, Sean Connery, David Niven, Peter Sellers, Terence Cooper, George Lazenby, Roger Moore, Timothy Dalton, Pierce Brosnan, and Daniel Craig

3. Barry Nelson gave his only appearance as James Bond in what Bond movie?
   The TV version of Casino Royale

4. Who played James Bond in On Her Majesty's Secret Service?
   George Lazenby

5. Who played James Bond on the 2006 movie Casino Royale?
   Daniel Craig

6. Pierce Brosnan played Bond on how many movies?
   4

7. Sean Connery played Bond on how many movies?
   7

8. Which Bond movie was Pierce Brosnan's debut at playing James Bond?
   GoldenEye

9. Roger Moore played Bond in how many movies?
   7

10. James Bond actor Pierce Brosnan also acted on what 2008 musical movie which starred Meryl Streep?
    Mamma Mia!

11. What was the name of the bad guy James Bond had to impersonate at the beginning of Octopussy?
    Colonel Luis Toro

12. Timothy Dalton played Bond on how many movies?
    2

13. David Niven gave his only appearance as Sir James Bond in what Bond movie?
    The comedy version of Casino Royale

14. What is a five letter word that describes James Bond perfectly?
    Suave

15. Pierce Brosnan played Bond in what 4 Bond movies?
    GoldenEye, Tomorrow Never Dies, The World Is Not Enough, and Die Another Day

16. Timothy Dalton played James Bond in what 2 Bond movies?
    The Living Daylights and Licence to Kill

17. Who played James Bond on the 1954 TV play Casino Royale?
    Barry Nelson

18. What are the 7 Bond movies Sean Connery starred in?
    Dr. No, From Russia with Love, Goldfinger, Thunderball, You Only Live Twice, Diamonds Are Forever, and Never Say Never Again

19. What are the 7 Bond movies Roger Moore starred in?
    Live and Let Die, The Man with the Golden Gun, The Spy Who Loved Me, Moonraker, For Your Eyes Only, Octopussy, and A View to a Kill

20. George Lazenby gave his only appearance as James Bond in which Bond movie?
    On Her Majesty's Secret Service

21. So far Daniel Craig played Bond in which 4 movies?
    Casino Royale (2006), Quantum of Solace, Skyfall, and SPECTRE

22. Peter Sellers played baccarat expert Evelyn Tremble who ends up posing as James Bond to confront Le Chiffre in what Bond movie?
    The comedy version of Casino Royale

23. Terence Cooper played Cooper who poses as James Bond in what Bond movie?
    The comedy version of Casino Royale

24. Which 2 Bond actors are on 7 James Bond movies?
    Sean Connery and Roger Moore

25. What is Sean Connery's middle name?
    Sean

26. What is Sean Connery's first name?
    Thomas

27. What is Roger Moore's middle name?
    George

28. What is George Lazenby's middle name?
    Robert

29. What is Pierce Brosnan's middle name?
    Brendan

30. What is Timothy Dalton's middle name?
    Peter

31. What is Daniel Craig's middle name?
    Wroughton

32. What 2 James Bond actors have birthdays in March?
    Daniel Craig and Timothy Dalton

33. Which James Bond actor would have been 91 on October 14, 2018?
    Roger Moore

34. Put the six main James Bond actors in order of age starting with the oldest.
    Roger Moore, Sean Connery, George Lazenby, Timothy Dalton, Pierce Brosnan, Daniel Craig

35. How does James Bond usually introduce himself?
    "The name is Bond. James Bond."

36. Besides James Bond 007 what name is James Bond also known as?
    Commander Bond

BOND GIRLS

1. What was the name of JIll St. John's character on Diamonds Are Forever?
   Tiffany Case

2. What was the name of Jane Seymour's character on Live and Let Die?
   Solitaire

3. Who played Lucia on the James Bond movie SPECTRE?
   Monica Bellucci

4. Who does James Bond team up with on The Spy Who Loved Me?
   Major Anya Amasova

5. On The Spy Who Loved Me what agent name was Major Anya Amasova also known as?
   Agent XXX

6. In On Her Majesty's Secret Service what does Tracy Vincenzo become at the end?
   Mrs. James Bond

7. Bond girl Sylvia Trench was on which 2 Bond movies?
   Dr. No and From Russia with Love

8. In On Her Majesty's Secret Service what was Tracy's formal name?
   Contessa Teresa de Vincenzo

9. What was the name of the main Bond girl on From Russia with Love?
   Tatiana Romanova

10. On Live and Let Die what was the name of the Bond girl who was working for Dr. Kananga?
    Rosie Carver

11. What was the name of the Bond girl played by Olga Kurylenko on the Bond movie Quantum of Solace?
    Camille

12. What was the name of the main Bond girl on Thunderball?
    Dominique Derval

13. On Goldfinger what was the name of the Bond girl who dies of skin suffocation while covered in gold paint?
    Jill Masterson

14. What was the name of the female cellist on The Living Daylights?
    Kara Milovy

15. Who plays Vesper Lynd on the 2006 Casino Royale?
    Eva Green

16. Who plays Vesper Lynd on the 1967 Casino Royale?
    Ursula Andress

17. On Goldfinger which Bond girl said, "I'm beginning to like you Mr. Bond?"
    Jill Masterson

18. Which Bond girl from which Bond movie said, "James. May I finally call you James?"
    Tiffany Case from Diamonds Are Forever

19. Who plays Tracy Vincenzo in On Her Majesty's Secret Service?
    Diana Rigg

20. On Thunderball what was Dominique Derval's nickname?
    Domino

21. Who played Domino Petachi on Never Say Never Again?
    Kim Basinger

22. Who played Octopussy in Octopussy?
    Maud Adams

23. Who played Andrea Anders on The Man with the Golden Gun?
    Maud Adams

24. On The World Is Not Enough what was the name of the Bond girl played by Denise Richards?
    Dr. Christmas Jones

25. Who played May Day on A View to a Kill?
    Grace Jones

26. What was the name of the new Bond girl who turned out to be the daughter of Mr. White on the Bond movie SPECTRE?
    Dr. Madeleine Swann

27. What was the name of the female secret agent on Skyfall who accidentally shot 007 off the train at the beginning and then at the end she takes the job as a secretary?
    Eve Moneypenny

28. What was the name of the main Bond girl on For Your Eyes Only?
    Melina Havelock

29. Actress Lea Seydoux played Dr. Madeleine Swann on the James Bond movie SPECTRE. Seydoux also played a female assassin on the fourth Mission: Impossible movie starring Tom Cruise. What was the name of the fourth Mission: Impossible movie?
    Mission: Impossible Ghost Protocol

30. What year was Maud Adams born?
    1945

31. What year was Honor Blackman born?
    1925

32. What year was Diana Rigg born?
    1938

33. On Die Another Day what was the name of Halle Berry's character?
    Jinx

WHICH JAMES BOND MOVIE...

1. The TV version of Casino Royale was the first James Bond movie ever made but what was the first James Bond movie that came out on the big screen?
   Dr. No

2. Which Bond movie was Geoffrey Keen's first time playing Frederick Gray?
   The Spy Who Loved Me

3. What Bond movie was a remake of the 1965 Bond movie Thunderball?
   Never Say Never Again

4. Which Bond movie was Geoffrey Keen's last time playing Frederick Gray?
   The Living Daylights

5. James Bond has an ally named Mathis on which 2 Bond movies?
   The 2006 version of Casino Royale and Quantum of Solace

6. Which Bond movie was Walter Gotell's last time playing General Gogol?
   The Living Daylights

7. Maud Adams was on which 2 Bond movies?
   The Man with the Golden Gun and Octopussy

8. Ursula Andress was on what 2 Bond movies?
   Dr. No and the 1967 version of Casino Royale

9. Which Bond movie won an Academy Award for Best Visual Effects?
   Thunderball

10. James Bond uses an Aston Martin Vanquish that can turn camouflage on which Bond movie?
    Die Another Day

11. James Bond swallows a tracking device capsule on which Bond movie?
    Thunderball

12. Which Bond movie has a part where James Bond is sitting in the car with the Bond girl and she almost shoots him?
    Quantum of Solace

13. Which Bond movie has a scene where James Bond and Zao are fighting each other in a clinic and Zao later runs out of the building and escapes on a helicopter while the Bond girl starts firing her gun at the helicopter?
    Die Another Day

14. Which Bond movie has a scene where James Bond is fighting bad guys in a hotel and on a hotel stairway?
    The 2006 version of Casino Royale

15. Which Bond movie has a scene where a bad guy puts a small bomb on a tanker truck out side the airport and while 007 and the bad guy are fighting each other in the truck 007 takes the bomb off the truck and sticks it to the bad guy's pants. When the bad guy is standing outside a police car dressed like a cop he sets off the bomb not knowing the bomb is sticking to his pants and he blows himself to death and James Bond 007 has a smile on his face?
    The 2006 version of Casino Royale

16. David Hedison played Felix Leiter on which 2 Bond movies?
    Live and Let Die and Licence to Kill

17. James Bond breaks into M's apartment to download information on which Bond movie?
    The 2006 version of Casino Royale

18. Which Bond movie has a part where 007's boss M has a man shoot a tracking device into Bond's forearm so they can keep a eye on Bond during his mission?
    The 2006 version of Casino Royale

19. Which James Bond movie has a part where James Bond kneels down to tie his shoes?
    The 2006 version of Casino Royale

20. Which Bond movie has a part where James Bond jumps off the back of a truck while chasing a bad guy?
    The 2006 version of Casino Royale

21. A gold ingot was used on which Bond movie?
    Goldfinger

22. The actor who played Mr. Ling on Goldfinger also acted on what 2 other Bond movies?
    You Only Live Twice and the comedy version of Casino Royale

23. Which Bond movie has a scene where James Bond leaves the villain in the middle of the desert with a can of oil?
    Quantum of Solace

24. Which James Bond movie has a scene where 007's friend Rene Mathis is killed by bad guys and James Bond dumps the body into the dumpster?
    Quantum of Solace

25. Which Bond movie has a scene where James Bond follows a bad guy into the BodyWorks exhibit?
    The 2006 version of Casino Royale

26. Can you name the James Bond movie where James Bond gets involved with a young woman who is seeking revenge for the murder of her parents and the bad guys are after a transmitter called the A.T.A.C. System?
For Your Eyes Only

27. Which James Bond movie has the part where the villain has the lady standing there with a cup of liquor on top of her head and then the bad guys try to force James Bond to shoot her but Bond misses as he fires the gun and the villain Raoul Silva shoots her dead?
Skyfall

28. Can you name the James Bond movie where 007 teams up with Agent XXX a.k.a. Major Anya Amasova and she's unaware that James Bond was the spy who killed her KGB boy friend in self defense?
The Spy Who Loved Me

29. James Bond has an ally named Valentin Zukovsky in which 2 Bond movies?
GoldenEye and The World Is Not Enough

30. Quarrel's son Quarrel Jr. helps James Bond on what movie?
Live and Let Die

31. Which 2 Bond movies had a character named Sheriff J.W. Pepper?
Live and Let Die and The Man with the Golden Gun

32. Which Bond movie was Robert Brown's first time playing M?
Octopussy

33. Which Bond movie was Robert Brown's last time playing M?
Licence to Kill

34. What Bond movie was Bernard Lee's first time playing M?
Dr. No

35. What Bond movie was Bernard Lee's last time playing M?
Moonraker

36. Can you name the James Bond movie where 007 tries to stop the villain from blowing up a bank in Fort Knox?
Goldfinger

37. Can you name the Bond movie where Commander John Strangways and his secretary are murdered by assassins who are known as the Three Blind Mice and 007 is sent to Jamaica to find out what happened to Strangways and James Bond meets Felix Leiter and Quarrel and the villain has his place in an island in Crab Key?
Dr. No

38. Which Bond movie has an ending where James Bond captures a bad guy named Mr. White?
The 2006 version of Casino Royale

39. Which James Bond movie has a scene where James Bond shows up in M's apartment to give her information?
The 2006 version of Casino Royale

40. Which Bond movie has a part where James Bond is lying down hooked up to machines and he fakes a cardiac arrest to check out?
Die Another Day

41. What James Bond movie has a finale where 007 goes through a funhouse maze through MI-6 to confront Blofeld and Blofeld sets the bomb for the building to blow up and 007 has to rescue Dr. Swann and to escape the building before it blows up?
SPECTRE

42. Which Bond movie has an action finale where James Bond and the Bond girl are in a plane full of enemies to stop the villain?
Die Another Day

43. Which Bond movie has a part where James Bond flips a bad guy off the motorcycle?
Quantum of Solace

44. Which Bond movie has a scene where James Bond is trying to escape from a S.W.A.T. team?
Quantum of Solace

45. Which Bond movie has an action scene where James Bond is battling bad guys in a building that has a fancy show going on?
Quantum of Solace

46. Which Bond movie has an action scene where James Bond is driving on the ice in a parachute firing vehicle and the villain uses his powerful satellite weapon to melt the ice James Bond is driving on?
Die Another Day

47. Which Bond movie has an action scene where James Bond is fighting bad guys on Hovercraft vehicles?
Die Another Day

48. Which Bond movie has James Bond using sunglasses that make him see himself battling enemies when he isn't in reality?
Die Another Day

49. Which Bond movie has a scene where James Bond and the villain fight each other with swords in a fencing place?
Die Another Day

50. Peter Sellers playing James Bond tries to defeat villain Orson Welles at baccarat on which James Bond movie?'
The comedy version of Casino Royale

51. Which James Bond movie has a scene where Sir James Bond is driving and he's being pursued by an enemy car and a remote control milk truck?
The comedy version of Casino Royale

52. What are the 6 James Bond movies that came out in the 80's?
For Your Eyes Only, Octopussy, Never Say Never Again, A View to a Kill, The Living Daylights, and Licence to Kill

53. What James Bond movie has a scene where James Bond is flying a little plane called Little Nellie and he starts getting pursued by enemy helicopters and Bond starts using his helicopter weapons?
You Only Live Twice

54. Which James Bond movie has an action scene where James Bond and Elektra King are skiing and they get pursued by enemies on parahawk vehicles?
The World Is Not Enough

55. Which James Bond movie has an action finale where James Bond and Christopher Walken are battling each other on top of the San Francisco Golden Gate Bridge?
A View to a Kill

56. Which James Bond movie has a scene where James Bond is in a circus tent disguised as a circus clown and he tries to defuse a bomb from blowing up?
Octopussy

57. Which James Bond movie has a scene where James Bond is battling bad guys in a ware house filled with fish, aquariums, and sharks?
Licence to Kill

58. What are the 7 James Bond movies that came out in the 60's?
Dr. No, From Russia with Love, Goldfinger, Thunderball, the comedy version of Casino Royale, You Only Live Twice, and On Her Majesty's Secret Service

59. Which James Bond movie has a scene where James Bond and Agent XXX are driving in a car and they get pursued by an enemy on a motorcycle, enemies in a car, and then an enemy in a helicopter and then James Bond drives the car into the ocean and transforms the car into a submarine car?
The Spy Who Loved Me

60. What are the 5 James Bond movies that came out in the 70's?
Diamonds Are Forever, Live and Let Die, The Man with the Golden Gun, The Spy Who Loved Me, and Moonraker

61. Which James Bond movie has a scene where James Bond is climbing a mountain to stop the bad guys and a bad guy up on the mountain tries to cause James Bond to fall off the mountain and James Bond uses his shoe laces to climb up the rope?
For Your Eyes Only

62. Which James Bond movie has a fight scene where James Bond is fighting bad guys on an ice hockey rink?
    For Your Eyes Only

63. Which James Bond movie has a scene where the villain has James Bond locked up in a cell and James Bond escapes through a tunnel and tries to stop the villain?
    Dr. No

64. Which James Bond movie has a part where James Bond fights 2 female bodyguards named Bambi and Thumper?
    Diamonds Are Forever

65. Which 1963 Bond movie starring Sean Connery was much later made as a PlayStation 2 video game in 2005?
    From Russia with Love

66. James Bond uses a fake leg cast at the end of which Bond movie?
    Octopussy

67. James Bond uses fake fingerprints on which Bond movie?
    Diamonds Are Forever

68. James Bond has Domino using a Geiger Counter camera on which Bond movie?
    Thunderball

69. James Bond uses a sea gull snorkel at the beginning of what Bond movie?
    Goldfinger

70. James Bond uses a manta ray disguise underwater on which Bond movie?
    Licence to Kill

71. What James Bond movie was Walter Gotell's first time playing General Alexis Gogol?
    The Spy Who Loved Me

72. James Bond uses an aerosol can on which Bond movie?
    Live and Let Die

73. James Bond uses an Avalanche Rescue Receiver at the beginning of which Bond movie?
    A View to a Kill

74. The actor who played Rodney on The Man with the Golden Gun had also played one of Morton Slumber's gangsters on what previous James Bond movie?
    Diamonds Are Forever

75. James Bond says he met his Waterloo on which Bond movie?
    The Living Daylights

76. A member of the S.P.E.C.T.R.E. organization talks about something called the British Train Robbery on which Bond movie?
Thunderball

77. Which Bond movie had a gypsy camp fight scene?
From Russia with Love

78. What Bond movie had bad guys putting a black widow spider in Bond's hotel room and shows a scene where Bond almost gets killed by the spider in bed?
Dr. No

79. Which Bond movie has a scene where Bond's ally Rene Mathis is arrested for being framed but later Mathis gets cleared before the end?
The 2006 version of Casino Royale

80. Pierce Brosnan's third Bond movie was The World Is Not Enough. Also the World Is Not Enough is known as the Bond family motto in what Bond movie?
On Her Majesty's Secret Service

81. Can you name the James Bond movie where the St. George's spy ship is sunk and James Bond gets involved with a young lady Melina Havelock as she seeks revenge for the murder of her parent while the bad guys are after a device called the A.T.A.C. System?
For Your Eyes Only

82. At the beginning of a Bond movie it showed James Bond putting flowers on his wife's grave and he soon gets on a helicopter and Blofeld gets control of the helicopter by remote control and Blofeld electrocutes the pilot and tries to kill Bond but Bond gets into the pilot's seat and later pulls the plug that has Blofeld's control of the helicopter and Blofeld no longer has control of the helicopter and now Bond has control of the helicopter and Bond flies the helicopter to Blofeld and Bond gets revenge against Blofeld for the murder of Mrs. James Bond which was back at the end of the Bond movie On Her Majesty's Secret Service. This brilliant beginning was the beginning of which Bond movie?
For Your Eyes Only

83. What James Bond movie has a quote where Ralph Fiennes as M says "A licence to kill is also a licence not to kill"?
SPECTRE

84. It never showed Blofeld's face in From Russia With Love. What other Bond movie in the 60's had Blofeld in it but never showed his face?
Thunderball

85. Which 2 Bond movies showed James Bond going to Shrublands Health Clinic?
Thunderball and Never Say Never Again

86. Blofeld had pets called Siamese fighting fish on what Bond movie?
From Russia with Love

87. Actor Charles Gray who played Dikko Henderson on You Only Live Twice also played Blofeld on what other Bond movie?
    Diamonds Are Forever

88. On the James Bond movies there's a crime organization called S.P.E.C.T.R.E. and the head of S.P.E.C.T.R.E. is a master criminal known as Ernst Stavro Blofeld. What are the 8 Bond movies that has Blofeld in it?
    From Russia with Love, Thunderball, You Only Live Twice, On Her Majesty's Secret Service, Diamonds Are Forever, For Your Eyes Only (at the beginning), Never Say Never Again, SPECTRE

89. Which 3 Bond movies had an action scene that had to do with a cable car?
    On Her Majesty's Secret Service, Moonraker, and SPECTRE

90. Actor Anthony Dawson played Professor Dent on Dr. No. Dawson had also played Blofeld on what 2 other Bond movies?
    From Russia with Love and Thunderball

91. Which Bond movie was Daniel Craig's second time playing Bond?
    Quantum of Solace

92. Which 2 Bond movies had an assassin named Jaws?
    The Spy Who Loved Me and Moonraker

93. The guy who played Kronsteen on From Russia with Love also acted on which version of Casino Royale?
    The 1967 version

94. Woody Allen played James Bond's evil nephew Jimmy Bond who turns out to be Dr. Noah the head of the crime organization called Smersh in what Bond movie?
    The comedy version of Casino Royale

95. Blofeld says to Bond, "I shall look forward personally to exterminating you Mr. Bond" on which Bond movie?
    You Only Live Twice

96. Blofeld said "That may not be convenient for some time" on which Bond movie?
    On Her Majesty's Secret Service

97. Blofeld says to Bond, "Nice to see you haven't lost that same mental edge 007" on which Bond movie?
    Diamonds Are Forever

98. James Bond said "See you in Miami" on which Bond movie?
    Octopussy

99. James Bond says "Switch the bloody machine off!" on which Bond movie?
    Licence to Kill

100. James Bond says "Thank God for hard currency!" on which Bond movie?
Octopussy

101. Blofeld says "A terrible catastrophe now confronts you!" on which Bond movie?
Never Say Never Again

102. James Bond uses the saying " They will be too bloody late" on which James Bond movie?
Skyfall

103. James Bond says "Next time I'm taking the elevator" on which Bond movie?
Tomorrow Never Dies

104. James Bond said "Someone's left with his tail between his legs" on which Bond movie?
Diamonds Are Forever

105. Can you name the James Bond movie where an enemy Russian agent Sergei Borzov tries to kill 007 on a mission and James Bond gets invo ved with his girlfriend Major Anya Amasova aka Agent XXX after James Bond kills her boyfriend in self defense and James Bond is on a mission to find out what happened to the nuclear submarines that are missing where 2 nuclear submarines were captured by the huge ship called the Liparus?
The Spy Who Loved Me

106. Can you name the Bond movie where the S.P.E.C.T.R.E. crime organization tries to set a death trap for 007 and James Bond goes to Istanbul to meet up with Ali Kerim Bey head of Station Turkey and James Bond is about to meet Tatiana Romanova who is trying to defect and James Bond is gonna steal from the consulate the Lektor decoding machine and they're gonna try to get away on a train?
From Russia with Love

107. Can you name the Bond movie where James Bond gets involved with a millionaire who loves Gold and tries to use a bomb to blow up a bank in Fort Knox and the villain has a butler named Oddjob who throws his steel hat as a weapon and James Bond has an Aston Martin DB5 filled with gadgets and weapons and a passenger ejector seat and the villain calls his scheme Operation Grand Slam?
Goldfinger

108. Can you name the James Bond movie where James Bond kills a S.P.E.C.T.R.E. agent disguised as a widow and then S.P.E.C.T.R.E. is up to Emilio Largo's NATO Project where Largo has Domino's brother killed and has Mr. Angelo look like Domino's brother through plastic operations and has the Air Force Plane the Vulcan stolen so the 2 atomic bombs will end in the hands of Largo and his men and James Bond goes to Shrubland Health Clinic and a S.P.E.C.T.R.E. agent tries to kill Bond and later the British Secret Service finds out about the stealing of the bombs and James Bond goes on a mission in Nassau?
Thunderball

109. Can you name the James Bond movie where 007 impersonates Colonel Luis Taro at the beginning and tries to get away on a mini jet and the bad guys send a missile to chase Bond but he outsmarts them and the missile blows up the bad guys warehouse and later 009 the British agent 009 disguised as a circus clown is killed by assassins from stealing

the Faberge egg and James Bond is sent on Operation Trobe where he finds Kamal Khan bidding for the Faberge egg at the auction and James Bond is on an adventure where he meets the woman on The Floating Palace who leads an Octopus cult and the bad guys attempt to blow up a U.S. Air Force Base in a circus and James Bond has to disguise himself as a circus clown to disarm the bomb in a circus tent after Kamal Khan and General Orlov take the jewelry out of the train?

Octopussy

110. Can you name the James Bond movie where Commander John Strangways gets shot and killed in Jamaica by three assassins known as the Three Blind Mice and they also shot and killed Strangways secretary and James Bond goes on a mission to Jamaica where 007 meets Felix Leiter and Quarrel. 007 survives an encounter with a black widow spider that the enemies put in his hotel room. A bad guy takes cyanide instead of telling 007 who he works for and the villain has a dragon tank in the Crab Key island to kill trespassers where the villain has a building where he's up to no good and 007 gets involved with a young lady in a white bikini and that lady was played by Ursula Andress and Joseph Wiseman plays the villain with steel hands. Jack Lord plays Felix Leiter the C.I.A. agent and Bernard Lee as 007's boss has Major Boothroyd switch James Bond's Beretta pistol with a Walther PPK?

Dr. No

111. Marc Forster directed the new Winnie the Pooh movie Christopher Robin. Marc Forster also directed Daniel Craig's second James Bond movie. What was Daniel Craig's second James Bond movie?

Quantum of Solace

ACTORS

1. Who played the new Blofeld on the James Bond SPECTRE?
   Christoph Waltz

2. Who played Felix Leiter on Dr. No?
   Jack Lord

3. Who played M on Never Say Never Again?
   Edward Fox

4. The actor who played Kronsteen on From Russia with Love had also played which character in the comedy version of Casino Royale?
   Le Chiffre's auctioneer

5. Who played Major Boothroyd on Dr. No?
   Peter Burton

6. Actor Walter Gotell who played General Gogol on the Bond movies also played which character on the Bond movie From Russia with Love?
   Morzeny

7. The actor who played Brad Whitaker on The Living Daylights also played which character on GoldenEye and Tomorrow Never Dies?
   Jack Wade

8. Who played Q on the 1967 Casino Royale?
   Geoffrey Bayldon

9. Who played Q Algernon in Never Say Never Again?
   Alec McCowen

10. On Licence to Kill what was the name of the drug runner who works for Sanchez?
    Milton Krest

11. On A View to a Kill what was the name of Max Zorin's head of security?
    Scarpine

12. On A View to a Kill what was Dr. Carl Mortner's name in actuality?
    Hans Glaub

13. Actor Jack Lord who played Felix Leiter on Dr. No is known for acting on what TV series?
    Hawaii Five-O

14. Who played Kerim Bey on From Russia with Love?
    Pedro Armendariz

15. John Huston played M on the 1967 Casino Royale. He was also one of the 5 directors of the movie. John Huston was the son of what actor?
    Walter Huston

16. Who played Willard Whyte on Diamonds Are Forever?
    Jimmy Dean

17. On Never Say Never Again Felix Leiter was played by what former football player?
    Bernie Casey

18. Name the actor who played the new Q on the two new James Bond movies Skyfall and SPECTRE.
    Ben Whishaw

19. Who played Kamal Khan on Octopussy?
    Louis Jourdan

20. Who played M on the 1967 James Bond comedy Casino Royale?
    John Huston

21. Who played Red Grant on From Russia with Love?
    Robert Shaw

22. Who played Professor Joe Butcher on Licence to Kill?
    Wayne Newton

23. Who played James Bond's nephew Jimmy Bond who turns out to be Dr. Noah the head of Smersh on the 1967 James Bond comedy Casino Royale?
    Woody Allen

24. Who played Le Chiffre on the 1967 James Bond comedy Casino Royale?
    Orson Welles

25. What were the names of the 2 twin brother actors who played Mischka and Grischka on Octopussy?
    David and Anthony Meyer

26. Actor Walter Gotell played General Gogol on more than one Bond movie. Gotell also played Morzeny in From Russia with Love before or after he played General Gogol?
    Before he played General Gogol

27. Actor Herve Villechaize played Nick Nack on The Man with the Golden Gun. Villechaize was also known for acting on what TV sitcom?
    Fantasy Island

28. Actor Desmond Llewelyn played Q on 17 James Bond movies. Llewellyn had also appeared on what Dick Van Dyke musical that was loosely based on a children's book by James Bond's creator Ian Fleming?
    Chitty Chitty Bang Bang

29. Actor Burt Kwouk played Mr. Ling on the third James Bond movie Goldfinger and he also played an auction man on the comedy version of Casino Royale and he also played a SPECTRE technician on the fifth James Bond movie You Only Live Twice. Burt Kwouk also played Clouseau's manservant who would always jump out at Inspector Jacques Clouseau on the Pink Panther movies. What was the name of Burt Kwouk's character on the Pink Panther movies?

    Cato

30. Who was the first actor to play M on the Bond movies?

    Bernard Lee

31. On the 1967 Casino Royale Jean-Paul Belmondo made a cameo before the end just like George Raft did. What was Belmondo's cameo role?

    The French Legionnaire

32. Actor Joe Don Baker who played Brad Whitaker on The Living Daylights also played which character on GoldenEye and Tomorrow Never Dies?

    Jack Wade

THE LADIES
(Some may be considered Bond Girls)

1. On Never Say Never Again what was the name of the female agent who works with Bond and gets killed by Fatima Blush?
   Nicole

2. On Thunderball what was the name of the female agent working with Bond and gives her life to protect Bond's mission?
   Paula Caplan

3. On Goldfinger what was the name of JIll Masterson's sister who seeks revenge against Goldfinger for the murder of Jill?
   Tilly Masterson

4. What was the name of the female S.P.E.C.T.R.E. agent on Thunderball?
   Fiona Volpe

5. On You Only Live Twice what was the name of the female S.P.E.C.T.R.E. agent who works with Mr. Osato?
   Helga Brandt

6. On The Man with the Golden Gun what was the name of Sheriff J.W. Pepper's wife?
   Mabel

7. On Dr. No what were the names of the 2 receptionists who work for Dr. No?
   Sister Rose and Sister Lily

8. On Dr. No which bad lady was played by Margaret LeWars?
   The photographer

9. Who played Rosa Klebb in From Russia with Love?
   Lotte Lenya

10. On the 1967 Casino Royale what was the name of the SMERSH agent who poses as M's daughter?
    Buttercup

11. On the 1967 Casino Royale what did agent Mimi pretend her name was?
    Lady Fiona

12. On The Spy Who Loved me what was the name of Karl Stromberg's assistant and helicopter pilot?
    Naomi

13. On Die Another Day what was the name of the lady who betrays Bond?
    Miranda Frost

14. On the 1967 Casino Royale what was the name of James Bond's late lover that the movie never showed?
    Mata Hari

15. Actress Martine Beswick played Paula Caplan on Thunderball. Beswick also played one of the gypsy camp fighting girls on what previous James Bond movie?
    From Russia with Love

16. The actress who played Bonita at the beginning of Goldfinger had also played Kerim Bey's girlfriend on what previous James Bond movie?
    From Russia with Love

17. On the 1967 Casino Royale what was the name of Mata Hari's dance teacher?
    Frau Hoffner

18. On Diamonds Are Forever what was the name of the older teacher who was involved with the diamond smuggling and gets murdered by Mr. Wint and Mr. Kidd?
    Mrs. Whistler

19. On Live and Let Die what was the name of the older flying student?
    Mrs. Bell

20. What was the name of the physical therapist at Shrublands Health Clinic on Thunderball and Never Say Never Again?
    Patricia Fearing

21. Joanna Pettet played James Bond's grown daughter Mata Bond in what Bond movie?
    The comedy version of Casino Royale

22. What was the name of the female dancer at the beginning of Goldfinger?
    Bonita

23. What was the name of the sinister SPECTRE agent on From Russia with Love?
    Rosa Klebb

24. On For Your Eyes Only what was the name of Bibi Dahl's figure skating teacher?
    Jacoba Brink

25. On the Bond movie On Her Majesty's Secret Service what was the name of the allergy patient who had an allergy to chickens?
    Ruby Bartlett

26. On the Bond movie On Her Majesty's Secret Service what was the name of the allergy patient who had an allergy to potatoes?
    Nancy

27. Samantha Bond played Moneypenny on how many Bond movies?
4

28. Who played Miss Moneypenny on Never Say Never Again?
Pamela Salem

29. Caroline Bliss played Miss Moneypenny on how many Bond movies?
2

30. Who played Miss Moneypenny on the 1967 James Bond comedy Casino Royale?
Barbara Bouchet

31. Who was the first actress to play Miss Moneypenny on the Bond movies?
Lois Maxwell

32. What is Miss Moneypenny's first name in the old Bond movies?
Gertrude

33. What is Miss Moneypenny's first name in the movies SPECTRE and Skyfall?
Eve

34. Which Bond movie was Lois Maxwell's first time playing Miss Moneypenny?
Dr. No

35. Which Bond movie was Lois Maxwell's last time playing Miss Moneypenny?
A View to a Kill

36. Who was the only actress to play M on the Bond movies?
Judi Dench

37. Judi Dench played M on how many Bond movies?
8

38. On GoldenEye what insult was M also known as?
The Evil Queen of Numbers

39. What was the name of Felix Leiter's wife on Licence to Kill?
Della Churchill

40. On Licence to Kill Della Churchill was played by what "Three's Company" star?
Priscilla Barnes

41. What was the name of the murderous lady on Never Say Never Again?
Fatima Blush

42. Who played Agent Mimi on the 1967 James Bond comedy Casino Royale?
Deborah Kerr

43. What was the name of Pleydell Smith's secretary who works for Dr. No?
    Miss Taro

44. Madonna sang the theme to Die Another Day. She also played which character on Die Another Day?
    Verity

45. The actress who played Ruby Bartlett in On Her Majesty's Secret Service also played Buttercup in what previous Bond movie?
    The comedy version of Casino Royale

46. What was the name of Max Zorin's girlfriend on A View to a Kill?
    May Day

47. What was the name of Blofeld's personal secretary in On Her Majesty's Secret Service?
    Fraulein Irma Bunt

48. On Tomorrow Never Dies what was the name of Elliot Carver's wife who used to be a girlfriend of Bond's?
    Paris Carver

NAMES

1. On The Living Daylights what was General Pushkin's full name?
   General Leonid Pushkin

2. On Never Say Never Again what was the name of Domino's rich boyfriend?
   Maximillian Largo

3. On Never Say Never Again what was the name of S.P.E.C.T.R.E.'s obedient servant?
   Captain Jack Petachi

4. What was the name of Electra King's father on The World Is Not Enough?
   Sir Robert King

5. On The World Is Not Enough the Bull was the name of Zukovsky's henchman. What was the Bull also known as?
   Bullion

6. What was the French title Blofeld tries to claim in on Her Majesty's Secret Service?
   Count Balthazar De Bleuchamp

7. In On Her Majesty's Secret Service Draco is head of what two companies?
   Draco Construction and The Union Course

8. In On Her Majesty's Secret Service what was the name of Blofeld's allergy clinic on Piz Gloria?
   Bleuchamp Institute of Allergy Research

9. What is the name of where James Bond works?
   British Secret Service

10. What is another name for where James Bond works?
    Her Majesty's Secret Service

11. What was the name of M's son on the 1967 Casino Royale?
    Hadley

12. On The Spy Who Loved Me what was Atlantis also known as?
    Stromberg Marine Research Laboratory

13. On Thunderball a motorized traction table was used to stretch a patient's spine. What was it called?
    The Rack

14. In On Her Majesty's Secret Service what was the name of the Swiss lawyer?
    Gebruder Gumbold

15. On the James Bond movies what was the name of James Bond's boss?
    M

16. On the Bond movie Quantum of Solace Mr. Greene was a member of what organization?
    Quantum

17. On the Bond movies there's a crime organization called S.P.E.C.T.R.E. What does S.P.E.C.T.R.E. stand for?
    Special Executive for Counter Intelligence, Terrorism, Revenge and Extortion

18. On The World Is Not Enough what was the name of the fellow Q was grooming for his replacement?
    R

19. On Never Say Never Again what name was Q also known as?
    Algernon

20. What was the name of Ralph Fiennes's character that replaces Judi Dench as the new M on the two new Bond movies Skyfall and SPECTRE?
    Gareth Mallory

21. On Licence to Kill what does Ed Killifer call his old friend Felix Leiter?
    Old Buddy

22. On the 1967 James Bond comedy Casino Royale what was the name of William Holden's character?
    Ransome

23. On the 1967 James Bond comedy Casino Royale what was M's other name?
    McTarry

24. On Goldfinger what was the brand name of the golf ball Goldfinger uses when he was playing golf with James Bond?
    Slazenger One

25. On Goldfinger what was the brand name of the golf ball that James Bond found when he was playing golf with Goldfinger?
    Slazenger Seven

26. What was the name of the machine on From Russia with Love?
    Lektor Decoding Machine

27. In On Her Majesty's Secret Service what does Blofeld call his female allergy patients?
    His own special angels of death

28. What was the name of Robert Brown's character on The Spy Who Loved Me?
    Admiral Hargreaves

29. On Dr. No what was Mr. Strangways full name?
    Commander John Strangways

30. What's the name of M's secretary?
    Miss Moneypenny

31. What was the name of James Bond's late wife from On Her Majesty's Secret Service?
    Tracy Vincenzo

32. On the 1967 Casino Royale what was Mata Bond's Indian title?
    Celestial Virgin of the Sacred Altar

33. What was Ian Fleming's middle name?
    Lancaster

34. On Moonraker when Bond was in Hugo Drax's centrifuge trainer what was the name of the button Bond had to press if the pressure was too much?
    The Chicken Switch

35. On Die Another Day what was the name of Gustav Graves satellite that reflects the sun's light?
    Icarus

36. On Never Say Never Again what was Q Algernon's nickname?
    Algy

37. At the beginning of Thunderball what was the name of the S.P.E.C.T.R.E. agent who faked his death?
    Colonel Jacques Boitier (Pronounced Bouvar)

38. What is the other name Q is also known for on the Bond movies?
    Q Branch

39. On Goldfinger what was the name of Goldfinger's henchman who gets killed by Oddjob at Fort Knox?
    Kisch

40. What was the name of Q's assistant on Octopussy?
    Smithers

41. On Goldfinger what was the name of Richard Vernon's character?
    Colonel Smithers

42. What was the name of the DEA agent who betrays Leiter on Licence to Kill?
    Ed Killifer

43. On Thunderball what was the name of Domino's murdered brother?
    Major Francois Derval

44. On Thunderball what was the name of the S.P.E.C.T.R.E. agent who looks just like Major Derval due to plastic surgery?
   Angelo Palazzi

45. On The Spy Who Loved Me what was the name of Anya's boyfriend who Bond kills in self defense?
   Sergei Barsov

46. What is the name of Bond's CIA ally on GoldenEye and Tomorrow Never Dies?
   Jack Wade

47. On Thunderball what was the name of Largo's ally who escapes with Bond and Domino when the Disco Volante was going to crash on the shore?
   Ladislav Kutze

48. What was the name of Colonel Moon's father on Die Another Day?
   General Moon

49. What was the name of Electra King's bodyguard on The World Is Not Enough?
   Gabor

50. What was the name of the Russian crime boss who helps Bond on GoldenEye and The World Is Not Enough?
   Valentin Zukovsky

51. In On Her Majesty's Secret Service what was the name of the guy James Bond was pretending to be to get to Blofeld?
   Sir Hilary Bray

52. What was the name of the fisherman who worked with Bond on Dr. No?
   Quarrel

53. What was the name of Tracy's father in On Her Majesty's Secret Service?
   Marc Ange Draco

54. On You Only Live Twice what was the name of Bond's ally who got killed by a bad guy?
   Dikko Henderson

55. What was the name of the Japanese Industrialist on You Only Live Twice?
   Mr. Osato

56. On the 1967 Casino Royale what was the name of the mysterious head of Smersh?
   Dr. Noah

57. On A View to a Kill what did James Bond pretend his name was to get to Max Zorin?
   James St. John Smythe

58. On From Russia with Love what was the name of the S.P.E.C.T.R.E. agent who was also a chessmaster?
Kronsteen

59. On Diamonds Are Forever what was the name of the cranky bad guy who works as a comedian?
Shady Tree

60. On For Your Eyes Only what was the name of the guy with the mustache who helps Bond?
Milos Columbo

61. On GoldenEye what was General Ourumov's full name?
General Arkady Grigorovich Ourumov

62. On GoldenEye what was Miskin's full name?
Defense Minister Dimitri Mishkin

63. What insult was 007's boss known for on the James Bond movie Thunderball that Miss Moneypenny refers to him?
The Old Man

64. On the 2012 James Bond movie Skyfall what nickname was Judi Dench as M also called?
Mom

65. On the 1967 Casino Royale what was the name of the other agent who poses as James Bond?
Cooper

66. In On Her Majesty's Secret Service what full name was Sir Hilary Bray also known as?
Sir Hilary Bray Baronet

67. In On Her Majesty's Secret Service what was the name of the British agent who helps Bond in Switzerland?
Campbell

68. On From Russia with Love what was Red Grant's first name?
Donald

69. What was the name of the bad guy James Bond impersonates on Diamonds Are Forever?
Peter Franks

70. On the 1967 Casino Royale what was the name of the officer who helps out Evelyn Tremble with his mission?
Lt. Mathis

71. On From Russia with Love what was the name of the agent Red Grant kills and impersonates to get to Bond?
Captain Nash

72. On From Russia with Love what does Red Grant keep calling Bond?
Old Man

73. What was the name of the radiation shield inspector on Diamonds Are Forever?
Klaus Hergesheimer

74. On Licence to Kill what was the name of Sanchez' head of security?
Heller

75. On The Spy Who Loved Me what was the name of the owner of the Mojaba Club?
Max Kalba

76. On A View to a Kill what did Bond pretend his name was when he met W.G. Howe?
James Stock

77. On The Man with the Golden Gun what was the name of the tough guy Bond had to fight in karate school?
Chula

78. What was the name of the person who was Scaramanga's sidekick on The Man with the Golden Gun?
Nick Nack

79. On The Man with the Golden Gun what was the name of the Asian industrialist Scaramanga works for?
Hai Fat

80. On Licence to Kill what was the name of the character who was played by Pedro Armendariz Jr?
President Hector Lopez

81. On the Bond movies what was General Gogol's first name?
Alexis

82. On the 1967 Casino Royale what was the name of Q's workshop assistant?
Fordise

83. On Tomorrow Never Dies what was the name of the tough bad guy working for Elliot Carver?
Stamper

84. On The Spy Who Loved Me what does Bond and Anya pretend their names are to get to Karl Stromberg?
Mr. and Mrs. Robert Sterling

85. On A View to a Kill what was the name of the British Secret Service agent who works undercover as James Bond's chauffeur?
Sir Godfrey Tibbett

86. On the 1967 Casino Royale after the credit sequence M and his men were being driven to Sir James Bond's mansion to pay the retired Sir James a visit. What were the names of the 3 men who were with M to visit Sir James?
    Ransome, Le Grand, and Smernov

87. On Live and Let Die what was the name of Sheriff J. W. Pepper's brother-in-law?
    Billy Bob

88. On Octopussy what was the name of the circus performer who flies out of the cannon?
    Francisco the Fearless

89. On From Russia with Love what does Bond and Tatiana Romanova pretend their name was when they were on the Orient Express?
    Mr. and Mrs. David Somerset

90. On The Man with the Golden Gun what was the name of Agent 002 who never appears on the movie?
    Bill Fairbanks

91. On For Your Eyes Only what was the name of the Chief of Staff who fills in for M while M was on leave?
    Tanner (Sometimes known as Bill Tanner)

92. What was the name of the multimillionaire on Diamonds Are Forever?
    Willard Whyte

93. On Live and Let Die what was the name of Mrs. Bell's flying trainer?
    Mr. Bleeker

94. On You Only Live Twice what was the name of Blofeld's bodyguard?
    Hans

95. On The Living Daylights what are the Afghan drug wholesalers known as?
    Snow Leopard Brotherhood

96. On From Russia with Love what was Kerim Bey's full name?
    Ali Kerim Bey

97. On Diamonds Are Forever what do Bond and Tiffany Case pretend their names are when they stay in the bridal suite at the Whyte House?
    Mr. and Mrs. Jones

98. On You Only Live Twice what did Bond pretend his name was to meet Mr. Osato?
    Mr. Fisher

99. On Octopussy what was the name of Kamal Khan's sidekick?
    Gobinda

100. What was the name of the creepy voodoo master on Live and Let Die?
Baron Samedi

GADGETS

1. What is the name of the inventor of Bond's gadgets?
   Q

2. What name is "Q" also known by?
   Major Boothroyd

3. James Bond uses a Mini Rebreather gadget underwater on Thunderball and the Mini rebreather later appeared in On Her Majesty's Secret Service. James Bond also used the Mini Rebreather underwater on which 2002 Bond movie?
   Die Another Day

4. In On Her Majesty's Secret Service when Bond breaks into Gumbold's office Bond uses a combination safe cracker to open the safe. What gadget went with the combination safe cracker?
   A printer

5. James Bond uses flash paper on which Bond movie?
   You Only Live Twice

6. James Bond uses a hairbrush transmitter on which Bond movie?
   Live and Let Die

7. James Bond and Alec Trevelyan use a code cracking device on which Bond movie?
   GoldenEye

8. James Bond uses a camera that he builds into a signature gun on which Bond movie?
   Licence to Kill

9. Bond and Blofeld use a voice simulator on which Bond movie?
   Diamonds Are Forever

10. James Bond uses a Visa card skeleton key on which Bond movie?
    The World Is Not Enough

11. James Bond uses a mobile phone with great gadgets on which Bond movie?
    Tomorrow Never Dies

12. James Bond uses a great key fob gadget on which 1987 Bond movie?
    The Living Daylights

13. Sir Godfrey Tibbett uses a shaver bug detector on which Bond movie?
    A View to a Kill

14. James Bond uses a bug detector on which 2 Bond movies?
    From Russia with Love and Live and Let Die

15. James Bond uses a briefcase bomb compartment on which Bond movie?
    Octopussy

16. James Bond uses a cheque copier gadget on which Bond movie?
    A View to a Kill

17. James Bond uses a wave walker gadget on which Bond movie?
    Diamonds Are Forever

18. James Bond uses Dentonite toothpaste and a cigarette package to blow and break the solid glass from Sanchez' meeting window on which Bond movie?
    Licence to Kill

19. Bond uses a ring camera gadget on which Bond movie?
    A View to a Kill

20. James Bond flies off a building by using a jetpack at the beginning of which Bond movie?
    Thunderball

21. James Bond uses a gadget called a book/tape recorder on which Bond movie?
    Thunderball

22. James Bond uses a binocular/monocular camera on which 2 Bond movies?
    For Your Eyes Only and GoldenEye

23. A laser camera was used on which Bond movie?
    Licence to Kill

24. James Bond uses an underwater camera on which Bond movie?
    Thunderball

25. Q uses a broom radio gadget on which Bond movie?
    Licence to Kill

26. On Thunderball what gadget does Largo use to open the door to the S.P.E.C.T.R.E. conference room?
    A cigarette case remote control

27. James Bond uses a gadget called a Geiger counter on which Bond movie?
    Dr. No

28. On Goldfinger James Bond puts a tracking device in Auric Goldfinger's car. Where does James Bond put a tracking device in later?
    In the heel of his shoe

29. On For Your Eyes Only what was the name of the gadget Bond and Q used for trying to identify the bad guy Bond needed to identify?
    Identigraph

30. On A View to a Kill what was the name of Q's doglike robot gadget that is also a video camera?
    Snooper

31. On You Only Live Twice Bond uses what kind of gadget to open Osato's safe?
    A pocket sized safe cracker

32. On Moonraker Bond carries a cigarette case that was also what kind of gadget?
    An X-ray safe cracker

33. On The Spy Who Loved Me what was the water gadget Bond drives on the water to get to Atlantis to get Anya out of there before the good guys on the submarine destroy Atlantis with torpedoes?
    Wet bike

34. On Moonraker when Bond takes the stuff out of Drax's safe what kind of cool gadget does James Bond use to photograph the stuff before putting the stuff back in the safe?
    A cigarette lighter camera

35. In On Her Majesty's Secret Service when James Bond is in Gumbold's office what kind of gadget does James Bond use to crack open the safe?
    A combination safe cracker

36. In On Her Majesty's Secret Service James Bond has his own cool spy camera that he uses on a great part in the movie. What does it say on the camera?
    I fooled you. It didn't say anything on the camera.

37. James Bond uses a sonic ring to break glass on which Bond movie?
    Die Another Day

MUSIC

1. Who sang the theme to the James Bond movie Skyfall?
   Adele

2. What Dusty Springfield song was on the 1967 Casino Royale?
   "The Look of Love"

3. The song "Nobody Does it Better" was the theme for the Bond movie The Spy Who Loved Me. Who sang the song?
   Carly Simon

4. At the beginning of A View to a Kill what Beach Boys song was playing when Bond was snow surfing away from the bad guys?
   "California Girls"

5. On the 1967 Casino Royale when Mata Bond opened the manhole to escape what song was coming from below the manhole?
   "What's New Pussycat?"

6. On Moonraker when Bond finds Drax's laboratory in Venice Bond had to press a few buttons that opened the door. The buttons he pressed played a musical tune which was a musical tune for aliens on what 1977 science fiction movie?
   Close Encounters of the Third Kind

7. On the 2007 season of American Idol which performer sang the theme to Diamonds Are Forever?
   Lakisha Jones

8. It showed frogs singing the theme for the Bond movie Live and Let Die at a frog funeral on what 2007 animated movie?
   Shrek the Third

9. Who sang the theme for Never Say Never Again?
   Lani Hall

10. What group sang the theme for A View to a Kill?
    Duran Duran

11. Who sang the theme to For Your Eyes Only?
    Sheena Easton

12. Who sang the theme to Thunderball?
    Tom Jones

13. Who sang the theme to From Russia with Love?
    Matt Monro

14. Who sang the theme for Goldfinger, Moonraker and Diamonds Are Forever?
    Shirley Bassey

15. On Octopussy the theme song for the movies was called "All Time High." Who sang the song?
    Rita Coolidge

16. Who sang the theme to Licence to Kill?
    Gladys Knight

17. Who sang the theme to You Only Live Twice?
    Nancy Sinatra

18. Who sang the theme to The Man with the Golden Gun?
    Lulu

19. Who sang the theme to Live and Let Die?
    Paul McCartney and Wings

20. Who sang the theme for Tomorrow Never Dies?
    Sheryl Crow

21. Who sang the theme for GoldenEye?
    Tina Turner

22. Who sang the theme for Die Another Day?
    Madonna

23. Who sang the song "Writing's on the Wall" that is the theme to the latest James Bond movie SPECTRE?
    Sam Smith

24. On The Living Daylights Miss Moneypenny is a fan of what singer?
    Barry Manilow

25. In On Her Majesty's Secret Service when a janitor was sweeping the janitor was whistling the theme for what Bond movie?
    Goldfinger

26. On the 1954 TV play Casino Royale when James Bond was playing the radio in his hotel suite the classical music on the radio was from what composer?
    Chopin

27. In On Her Majesty's Secret Service there was a song in the movie called "We Have All The Time in the World." Who sang the song?
    Louis Armstrong

28. The James Bond theme remix from Tomorrow Never Dies was done by whom?
    Moby

29. The James Bond theme mix by Moby starts out with the voice of Pierce Brosnan as James Bond. The song later plays the voices of what 2 actors?
    Sean Connery as James Bond and Gert Frobe as Goldfinger

30. On Dr. No at a Jamaican bar a guy was on stage singing. What song does he sing?
    "Jump Up Jamaica"

31. The theme song for the Bond movie Quantum of Solace was called "Another Way to Die." Who sang the song?
    Jack White and Alicia Keys

32. What band sang the theme for The Living Daylights?
    A-Ha

33. What music group composed the theme music for Dr. No?
    John Barry and Orchestra

34. Who sang the theme for The World Is Not Enough?
    Garbage

35. Which music group composed the theme music for On Her Majesty's Secret Service?
    The John Barry Orchestra

36. The theme song for the 2006 Casino Royale was called "You Know My Name." Who sang the song?
    Chris Cornell

37. The theme music for the 1967 Casino Royale was played by which two musicians?
    Herb Alpert and the Tijuana Brass, Burt Bacharach

38. What Christmas tune was being sung during the ice skating scene in On Her Majesty's Secret Service?
    "Do You Know How Christmas Trees Are Grown"

VILLAINS

1. Who played the villain Raoul Silva on the James Bond movie Skyfall?
   Javier Bardem

2. What was the name of the villain on The Man with the Golden Gun?
   Francisco Scaramanga

3. What was the name of Willard Whyte's right hand man and traitor on Diamonds Are Forever?
   Bert Saxby

4. At the beginning of The Man with the Golden Gun what was the name of the hitman who tries to take on Scaramanga?
   Rodney

5. What was the name of the villain on For Your Eyes Only?
   Aristotle Kristatos a.k.a. Aris Kristatos

6. On For Your Eyes Only what was the name of the brutal tough guy working for Kristatos?
   Eric Kriegler

7. On Live and Let Die what was the name of the soft voiced bad guy working for Dr. Kananga?
   Whisper

8. On Licence to Kill what was the name of the killer working for Sanchez?
   Dario

9. On For Your Eyes Only what was the name of the killer with the glasses?
   Emile Leopold Locque

10. What were the names of the 2 main villains on Die Another Day?
    Gustav Graves, Colonel Moon

11. What was the name of the villain on Tomorrow Never Dies?
    Elliot Carver

12. What was the name of the villain on A View to a Kill?
    Max Zorin

13. On Never Say Never Again what was the name of the bad guy with the beard who works with Largo on the Tears of Allah operation?
    Dr. Kovacs

14. On Die Another Day what was the name of the Asian bad guy who gets a diamond scar on his face?
    Zao

15. Who played Max Zorin on A View to a Kill?
    Christopher Walken

16. On Goldfinger what was the name of the gangster who gets shot by Oddjob in the car?
    Mr. Solo

17. On Goldfinger what was the name of the American gangster played by Bill Nagy?
    Mr. Midnight

18. On Goldfinger what was the name of the American gangster played by Hal Galili?
    Mr. Strap

19. What were the names of the 2 main villains on The World Is Not Enough?
    Victor Zokas a.k.a. Renard, Elektra King

20. On For Your Eyes Only what was the name of the Cuban hitman paid to kill Mr. and Mrs. Havelock?
    Hector Gonzales

21. On The World Is Not Enough what was the name of Valentin Zukovsky's henchman who was actually working for Renard?
    The Bull

22. Which villain on which Bond movie said "There is no news like bad news"?
    Elliot Carver from Tomorrow Never Dies

23. Who were the 2 characters who killed Bond's wife at the end of On Her Majesty's Secret Service?
    Ernst Stavro Blofeld and Fraulein Irma Bunt

24. On Never Say Never Again what was the name of the tough S.P.E.C.T.R.E. agent who tries to kill Bond at Shrublands Health Clinic?
    Lippe

25. On the 1954 TV play Casino Royale Le Chiffre has 3 henchmen. What were the names of his 3 henchmen?
    Basil, Zoltan, and Zuroff

26. On Thunderball what was the name of the memorable killer working for Largo?
    Vargas

27. Which villain from which Bond movie uses an inhaler?
    Le Chiffre from the 2006 version of Casino Royale

28. On For Your Eyes Only the villain's name was Aristotle Kristatos. What does Bibi Dahl call him?
    Uncle Ari

29. Which 3 Bond movies had a villain named Le Chiffre?
The 3 Bond movies called Casino Royale

30. What was the name of the evil general on GoldenEye?
General Ourumov

31. On The Living Daylights what was the name of the cold blooded killer working for Whittaker and Koskov?
Necros

32. On the 2006 Bond movie Casino Royale what was the name of the villain Le Chiffre was working for?
Mr. White

33. What was the name of the villain on GoldenEye?
Alec Trevelyan

34. What was the name of the villain on Licence to Kill?
Franz Sanchez

35. What was the name of the main villain on the Bond movie Quantum of Solace?
Dominic Greene

36. Which bad guy on which Bond movie has a mechanical arm from losing his arm to a crocodile?
Tee Hee from Live and Let Die

37. What were the names of the two twin assassins on Octopussy?
Mischka and Grischka

38. On For Your Eyes Only what was the name of the bad guy who tries to kill Bond on the cliff?
Apostis

39. On For Your Eyes Only what was the name of the bad guy who gets killed by Columbo's men at the beach?
Claus

40. On Goldfinger what was the name of the assassin sent by Ramirez to kill Bond?
Capungo

41. On Thunderball what was the name of the S.P.E.C.T.R.E. agent who tries to kill Bond at Shrublands Health Clinic?
Count Lippe

42. On From Russia with Love what was the name of the bad guy who kills for pleasure?
Krilencu

43. What were the names of the 2 main villains on The Living Daylights?
General Georgi Koskov and Brad Whittaker

44. What was the name of the villain on The Spy Who Loved Me?
Karl Stromberg

45. What was the name of the grinning killer on Live and Let Die?
Tee Hee

46. What was the name of the villain on Live and Let Die?
Dr. Kananga

47. What was the name of the villain on Moonraker?
Hugo Drax

48. What were the names of the 2 main villains on Octopussy?
Kamal Khan and General Orlov

49. On Octopussy the villain was after what kind of fancy thing?
A Faberge egg

50. Who is the head of the S.P.E.C.T.R.E organization?
Ernst Stavro Blofeld

51. On Dr. No what was Dr. No's first name?
Julius

52. In From Russia with Love what was the name of the S.P.E.C.T.R.E. agent in charge of SPECTRE Island?
Morzeny

53. What was the name of the computer programmer with glasses on GoldenEye?
Boris Grishenko

54. What was the name of Goldfinger's mute sidekick on Goldfinger?
Oddjob

55. On Diamonds Are Forever what was the name of the bad guy who runs a funeral home?
Morton Slumber

56. On Moonraker what was the name of Hugo Drax's Asian bodyguard?
Chang

57. On the Bond movie On Her Majesty's Secret Service what was the name of the thug working for Blofeld?
Grunther

58. On Dr. No what was the name of Dr. No's spymaster?
Professor R.J. Dent

59. On Goldfinger what was the name of the Chinese man who works with Goldfinger in Operation Grand Slam?
    Mr. Ling

60. On Live and Let Die what was the name of Dr. Kananga's second identity?
    Mr. Big

61. On Diamonds Are Forever what were the names of the 2 goofball killers working for Blofeld?
    Mr. Wint and Mr. Kidd

62. On Dr. No what was the name of the bad guy who poses as a chauffeur?
    Mr. Jones

63. On Licence to Kill what was the name of the bad guy who was a financial wizard?
    William Truman-Lodge

64. On The Spy Who Loved Me what was the name of the bad guy who gets killed by Jaws at the pyramids?
    Aziz Fekkesh

65. On Dr. No there were three killers who pretend to be blind men. What were those three killers known as?
    The Three Blind Mice

66. Who played Dr. No on Dr. No?
    Joseph Wiseman

67. Who played Jaws on The Spy Who Loved Me and Moonraker?
    Richard Kiel

68. Who played Blofeld on Never Say Never Again?
    Max Von Sydow

69. Who played Le Chiffre on the 2006 Casino Royale?
    Mads Mikkelsen

70. Who played Blofeld in On Her Majesty's Secret Service?
    Telly Savalas

71. Who played Blofeld on You Only Live Twice?
    Donald Pleasence

72. Who played Blofeld on Diamonds Are Forever?
    Charles Gray

UNPLEASANT DEMISES

1. On The World Is Not Enough which character kills Mr. Lachaise and Sir Robert King and later commits suicide on a hot air balloon?
   The cigar girl

2. On From Russia with Love what kind of special weapon does Rosa Klebb use before the end?
   A shoe with a poisonous knife at the end

3. On From Russia with Love how does Kerim Bey die?
   Kerim Bey and Benz get killed by Red Grant on the Orient Express. When Bond finds the 2 bodies on the floor it looked like they obviously killed each other.

4. What was the last name of the character who was murdered at the beginning of Dr. No?
   Strangways

5. In On Her Majesty's Secret Service what was the name of the germ-warfare virus that Blofeld plans to spread if his demands are not met?
   Virus Omega

6. On A View to a Kill how does Max Zorin die?
   Zorin and Bond were fighting each other on top of the San Francisco Golden Gate Bridge and Zorin fell off the bridge.

7. On Licence to Kill what was the name of the bad guy who kills Heller with a forklift blade?
   Braun

8. On Live and Let Die what was the name of the bad guy who gets killed in an explosion while pursuing Bond in a speedboat?
   Adam

9. On For Your Eyes Only what was the name of Melina Havelock's murdered father?
   Sir Timothy Havelock

10. On The World Is Not Enough how was Renard slowly dying?
    He had a bullet in his head.

11. On For Your Eyes Only Emile Locque leaves what kind of pin on Ferrara's corpse?
    A dove pin

12. On You Only Live Twice Blofeld has what kind of dead y pets?
    Piranha fish

13. On the James Bond movie Dr. No when James Bond and the villain Doctor No are fighting each other in the control room, James Bond climbs back up to safety but Doctor No's steel hands were not for climbing and Doctor No drowns into the boiling liquid. What happens next?
    James Bond has to find Ursula Andress and they have to escape from the facility before it blows up.

14. On For Your Eyes Only what was the name of Bond's ally who gets killed by Emile Locque?
    Luigi Ferrara

15. On the James Bond movie For Your Eyes Only when Melina Havelock is seeking to kill Aris Kristatos for the murder of her parents James Bond says "no Melina. That's not the answer. We'll turn him over to the Greek police." When they're not looking Kristatos takes out his knife and was about to kill them. What happens next?
    James Bond's ally Milos Columbo throws a knife on Kristatos' back, killed Kristatos and saved Jame Bond and Melina Havelock's lives.

16. On the James Bond movie Thunderball James Bond and Emilio Largo are fighting each other on The Disco Volante yacht and Largo picks up Bond's gun. Largo was about to shoot him but Domino shoots Largo in the back with an underwater harpoon gun to save Bond's life and to avenge the death of her brother Francois. What happens next?
    Domino says to James Bond that she's glad she killed him and then James Bond says, "You're glad?"

MISSIONS & PLOTS

1. What was James Bond's mission on the 1954 TV play Casino Royale?
   To defeat Le Chiffre at baccarat

2. On Never Say Never Again what was the name of S.P.E.C.T.R.E.'s operation?
   The Tears of Allah

3. On You Only Live Twice the S.P.E.C.T.R.E. rocket was called Intruder. What was the Rocket's code name on its final mission?
   Bird One

4. On For Your Eyes Only what was the name of Bond's mission to recover the A.T.A.C. System?
   Operation Undertow

5. On Goldfinger what was the name of Mr. Goldfinger's plot to have planes spray nerve gas to make the town fall asleep?
   Operation Rock A Bye Baby

6. In Octopussy what was the name of Bond's mission to discover who was selling the Faberge Egg?
   Operation Trove

7. On Diamonds Are Forever Bond and the CIA had an operation. What was that operation called?
   Operation Passover

8. On the Bond movie On Her Majesty's Secret Service what was the name of Bond's operation to search for Blofeld?
   Operation Bedlam

9. On A View to a Kill what was the codename for Zorin's evil plot?
   Project Main Strike

10. On Goldfinger what was the name of Goldfinger's villa nous plot?
    Operation Grand Slam

11. What was S.P.E.C.T.R.E.'s mission on From Russia with Love?
    To lure James Bond to his death

12. On Thunderball what was the codename for S.P.E.C.T.R.E.'s scheme?
    NATO Project

13. On Goldfinger what were the principal ingredients that Auric Goldfinger uses for the bomb on operation Grand Slam?
    Cobalt and iodine

14. In On Her Majesty's Secret Service what was the code phrase for the helicopter attack on Piz Gloria where Bond, Draco and Draco's men rescue Tracy and destroy the Bleuchamp Institute?
    Demolition Deal

FOOD & DRINK

1. How does James Bond like his vodka martinis made?
   Shaken. Not stirred.

2. On For Your Eyes Only what does Milos Columbo love to eat?
   Pistachio nuts

3. On From Russia with Love what breakfast selection does Bond order on the phone in the bridal suite?
   Green figs, yogurt, coffee - very black

4. In On Her Majesty's Secret Service what was Bonds dinner entree when he had dinner with Fraulein Bunt and the female patients?
   Steak Piz Gloria

5. On Never Say Never Again when Bond was at Shrublands Health Clinic he smuggled his own food in his briefcase. What 4 types of food did he smuggle?
   Beluga caviar, quail's eggs, vodka, and foie gras from Strasbourg

6. On Goldfinger what was Mr. Goldfinger's favorite drink?
   Mint Julep

7. On the 1967 Casino Royale in the middle of the movie when Sir James Bond was retired what was his drink of choice?
   Jasmine tea

8. On Never Say Never Again when Bond is at Shrublands Health Clinic he gets served what 3 types of entrees?
   Lentil Delight, Dandelion Salad, and Goat's Cheese

9. On Dr. No when Bond is staying in Jamaica what kind of drink is brought to him by room service?
   Medium dry vodka martini, mixed, not stirred.

10. On You Only Live Twice when Dikko Henderson made Bond a vodka martini how was the martini made?
    Stirred, not shaken.

11. On The Man with the Golden Gun what was the name of the champagne served to Bond and Mary?
    Phuyuck

12. On You Only Live Twice right before Bond found Osato's safe what was the name of the drink Bond tries that he didn't like?
    Siamese vodka

13. On Never Say Never Again when Bond buys Domino Petachi a drink what drink does Bond order for himself?
    Vodka on the rocks

14. On Never Say Never Again when Bond buys Domino Petachi a drink what kind of drink does Domino order?
    Double Bloody Mary with plenty of Worcestershire sauce

15. What James Bond movie has the line where James Bond says that Peking duck is different from Russian caviar but he loves them both?
    You Only Live Twice

16. On Thunderball when Bond and Domino are at a table by the hotel pool what seafood entree does Bond eat?
    Conch chowder

17. In On Her Majesty's Secret Service what kind of breakfast selection does Bond order from Room Service?
    Cafe complait for two with fresh orange juice

18. On Goldfinger Mr. Ramirez uses what to finance revolutions?
    Drugs smuggled in heroin flavored bananas

19. On Never Say Never Again when M told Bond about the toxins that destroy the body and the brain what 3 things did M say cause those toxins in Bond's case?
    Too much red meat, white bread, and dry martinis

LOCATIONS

1. On Never Say Never Again what was the name of the place where Captain Jack Petachi works?
   Swadley Air Base

2. At the beginning of The Living Daylights where did the Double O agent training exercise take place?
   Gibraltar

3. On From Russia with Love Red Grant had escaped from where in 1960?
   Dartmoor Prison in England

4. On Thunderball what was the name of Emilio Largo's seaside Nassau estate?
   Palmyra

5. On Never Say Never Again what was the name of Max Largo's North African fortress estate?
   Palmyra

6. What was the name of the mountaintop where Blofeld's allergy clinic takes place in On Her Majesty's Secret Service?
   Piz Gloria

7. What was the name of Ian Fleming's beachfront vacation home in Jamaica?
   Goldeneye

8. In On Her Majesty's Secret Service Bond tries to talk Blofeld into going with him on a trip to where?
   Augsburg

9. On the 1954 TV play Casino Royale when James Bond gives Clarence Leiter Zoltan's cane where does Bond tell Clarence to put the cane?
   In Scotland Yard's Black Museum

10. In On Her Majesty's Secret Service Sir Hilary Bray is a heraldry specialist at what college?
    The London College of Arms

11. In On Her Majesty's Secret Service what do they call the room in Blofeld's allergy clinic were James Bond has dinner with Fraulein Bunt and Blofeld's allergy patients?
    The Alpine Room

12. On Dr. No what was the name of Dr. No's Island?
    Crab Key

13. On The Spy Who Loved Me what was the name of Stromberg's huge spider-like place that is sometimes underwater and sometimes not?
    Atlantis

TRANSPORTATION

1. On Thunderball what do they call the plane that carried 2 atomic bombs that were hijacked by S.P.E.C.T.R.E?
   The Vulcan

2. On Octopussy what was the name of Bond's cool mini jet he used at the beginning?
   Acrostar Mini Jet

3. What was the name of Milton Krest's ship on Licence to Kill?
   Wavekrest

4. What was the name of Largo's yacht on Never Say Never Again?
   The Flying Saucer

5. At the beginning of Octopussy what was the Acrostar Mini Jet also known as?
   Bede Jet

6. On For Your Eyes Only what was the name of the ship that had the A.T.A.C. system inside?
   St. Georges

7. On Diamonds Are Forever what was the name of Blofeld's one man submarine?
   Bathosub

8. On The Spy Who Loved Me what was the name of the huge ship that captured nuclear submarines?
   Liparus

9. James Bond uses a rocket powered flying motorcycle on which Bond movie?
   Never Say Never Again

10. On Thunderball what was the name of Largo's ship?
    The Disco Volante

11. On The Spy Who Loved Me what was the name of Bond's car that could transform into a submarine car?
    Lotus Esprit Submarine Car

12. On The Spy Who Loved Me what was the nickname of Bond's Lotus Esprit Submarine car?
    Wet Nellie

13. What was the name of the spacecraft abducted at the beginning of You Only Live Twice?
    Jupiter 16

14. On the 1967 James Bond comedy Casino Royale what did Evelyn Tremble call his cool looking fast car?
    His Lotus Formula Three

15. What kind of car is James Bond sometimes famous for driving?
    Aston Martin DB5

16. Besides Aston Martin DB5 what other Aston Martin does James Bond sometimes use?
    Aston Martin DBS

17. What kind of Aston Martin does Bond use on The Living Daylights?
    An Aston Martin V8 with a self destruct system

18. On Live and Let Die what was Whisper's white Cadillac known as?
    Pimpmobile

19. On For Your Eyes Only what was the name of Timothy Havelock's two men submarine?
    Neptune

20. What 2 Bond movies have excellent scenes with bobsleds?
    On Her Majesty's Secret Service and For Your Eyes Only

21. James Bond uses a crocodile submarine in what Bond movie?
    Octopussy

22. On Dr. No the bad guys in Crab Key use a fire blowing vehicle that looks like what fire breathing animal?
    A dragon

23. On Never Say Never Again what was the name of the rocket powered flying machines James Bond and Felix Leiter were using?
    XT 7B

24. What was the name of the S.P.E.C.T.R.E. rocket on You Only Live Twice?
    Intruder

25. James Bond uses a car with great gadgets including a passenger ejector seat on which Bond movie?
    Goldfinger

26. On Never Say Never Again when Bond discovers that female agent Nicole had been killed by Fatima Blush Fantima who starts running and gets away in her car. Bond goes after her in what cool vehicle gadget?
    A rocket powered motorcycle

WEAPONS a.k.a. INSTRUMENTS OF DEATH

1. On Moonraker when the good guys and the bad guys are battling each other in space what kind of guns were they shooting at each other with instead of regular guns?
   Laser guns

2. On Thunderball when Bond, the good guys, and the bad guys are battling each other underwater what kind of guns were they shooting at each other with instead of regular guns?
   Spear guns

3. On Dr. No what kind of gun does James Bond carry before M has Major Boothroyd switch Bond's gun to a Walther PPK?
   A Beretta pistol

4. On Never Say Never Again what was the name of the 2 nuclear warheads abducted by S.P.E.C.T.R.E.?
   W-80

5. On The Man with the Golden Gun what other special weapon does Scaramanga have besides his golden gun?
   Solar powered laser cannon

6. James Bond uses a finger clamp weapon at the beginning of which Bond movie?
   Diamonds Are Forever

7. On From Russia with Love what kind of special weapon does Red Grant carry?
   A wrist watch strangle wire

8. What was the scary weapon a thug carries on Octopussy?
   A buzz saw YoYo

9. On the 1954 TV play Casino Royale Zoltan carries his own secret weapon. What kind of weapon does Zoltan carry?
   A gun disguised as a cane

10. On the 1954 TV play Casino Royale Le Chiffre carries 3 razor blades for slashing purposes. Where does he carry those 3 razor blades?
    He carries one in his hat band, one in the heel of his left shoe and one in his cigarette case.

11. On Goldfinger what was the name of the nerve gas Mr. Goldfinger has used for Operation Grand Slam?
    Delta Nine

12. On For Your Eyes Only what device was the villain after?
    The A.T.A.C. System

13. James Bond has cigarettes that shoot out rocket powered darts on which Bond movie?
    You Only Live Twice

14. Bad guys use a weapon called a Laser Net on which Bond movie?
    Die Another Day

15. James Bond uses a pen gun that shoots out a rocket powered bullet on which Bond movie?
    Never Say Never Again

16. James Bond uses a pen grenade on which Bond movie?
    GoldenEye

17. On From Russia with Love what gadget of Bond's is James Bond able to build into a sniper rifle?
    Bond's top secret briefcase

18. A bad guy named Necros uses milk bottle grenades on which Bond movie?
    The Living Daylights

19. James Bond uses glasses detonator on which Bond movie?
    The World Is Not Enough

20. Blofeld uses a diamond satellite weapon for his evil plot on which Bond movie?
    Diamonds Are Forever

21. James Bond uses a wrist dart gun on which Bond movie?
    Moonraker

22. On Goldfinger what does Oddjob use as a weapon to throw at his enemies?
    His hat

23. On the 1967 Casino Royale Dr. Noah has his own pill that turns people into what?
    A walking time bomb

24. On The Living Daylights what was the name of the radio that shoots out a rocket?
    Ghetto Blaster

SIGNS & PASSWORDS & WHAT DID IT SAY?

1. On the 1967 Casino Royale during the casino fight scene a man in the casino calls the police and it shows the police running out of the police station and getting away on a vehicle. What did it say on the sign that was on the police station?
   Bonds

2. In On Her Majesty's Secret Service when Sir Hilary Bray showed Bond a paper of Bond's coat of arms what motto does it say for James Bond's coat of arms?
   The World Is Not Enough

3. On Moonraker when James Bond uses his cigarette lighter camera what does it say on his cigarette lighter camera?
   007

4. At the beginning of Dr. No what was the call sign for MI-7 communications headquarters?
   G7W

5. On the 1967 Casino Royale during the casino fight scene a dog is biting someone's clothing. What did it say on the dog's collar?
   007

6. On The Spy Who Loved Me when Bond found that Kalba had been murdered by Jaws by the phone booths what did it say on the sign Bond put on the corpse?
   OUT OF ORDER

7. On the 1967 Casino Royale during the great casino fight scene two walruses start fighting each other. Later both walruses are wearing a silver medal. What did it say on their silver medals?
   007

8. At the beginning of Dr. No what was the call sign for Mr. Strangeways' transmitter?
   W6N

9. On A View to a Kill what did it say on Max Zorin's blimp style airplane?
   Zorin Industries

10. On For Your Eyes Only what does A.T.A.C. stand for?
    Automatic Targeting Attack Communicator

11. In On Her Majesty's Secret Service when Draco and his chauffeur dropped off Bond to break into Gumbold's office what kind of billboard does it show on the background?
    A billboard for Camel cigarettes

12. On Goldfinger when Felix Leiter was trying to track down Bond on Bond's Homer Tracking Device what famous restaurant does it show on the background?
    Kentucky Fried Chicken

13. On Dr. No when James Bond enters Miss Moneypenny's office what does it say on the door of her office?
    Universal Exports

14. On You Only Live Twice after Bond faked his assassination what did it say on the newspaper about it?
    BRITISH NAVAL COMMANDER MURDERED

15. On Licence to Kill when Felix Leiter and his bride Della gave James Bond a gold cigarette lighter what did it say on the lighter?
    JAMES, LOVE ALWAYS. DELLA AND FELIX

16. On For Your Eyes Only when Tanner gave Bond a classified thing what did it say on the white ribbon that was wrapped around the classified thing?
    FOR YOUR EYES ONLY

17. On GoldenEye when Boris Grishenko is writing an email to the FBI what does he type on the email?
    Better Luck Next Time Slugheads.

18. On Thunderball what did it say on the 2 atomic bombs Largo and his men stole from the Vulcan?
    HANDLE LIKE EGGS

19. At the beginning of For Your Eyes Only when Bond puts flowers on his wife's grave what did it say on the grave?
    TERESA BOND
    1943 - 1969
    BELOVED WIFE OF JAMES BOND.
    WE HAVE ALL THE TIME IN THE WORLD.

20. On Licence to Kill after Sanchez and his men fed Felix Leiter to the sharks Bond later found Leiter alive. What did it say on the note Sanchez and his men left on Leiter?
    HE DISAGREED WITH SOMETHING THAT ATE HIM.

21. On Live and Let Die at Dr. Kananga's alligator farm what did it say on the gate?
    TRESPASSERS WILL BE EATEN.

22. On the preview for the 1967 Casino Royale what catch phrase did they use at the end of the preview?
    Join the Casino Royale Fun Movement

23. On Diamonds Are Forever what did it say on the cover for the cassette tape Blofeld uses for his evil plot?
    World's Greatest Marches

24. On You Only Live Twice what was the password between British Intelligence and Japanese S.I.S.?
    I Love You

25. On The World Is Not Enough what was Electra King's motto?
    There's no point in living if you can't feel alive.

26. On the 2006 version of Casino Royale James Bond had to make a password for the money. James Bond named the password after his gir friend. What was the password?
    Vesper

27. On From Russia with Love when Bond gives Miss Moneypenny a photo what did he write on the photo?
    From Russia With Love

DATES

1. The Bond movie Skyfall came out in what year?
   2012

2. The Bond movie On Her Majesty's Secret Service came out in what year?
   1969

3. The Bond movie Dr No came out in what year?
   1962

4. The Bond movie The Living Daylights came out in what year?
   1987

5. Live and Let Die came out in what year?
   1973

6. Diamonds Are Forever came out in what year?
   1971

7. From Russia with Love came out in what year?
   1963

8. Goldfinger came out in what year?
   1964

9. Which 2 Bond movies came out in 1967?
   You Only Live Twice and the comedy version of Casino Royale

10. Thunderball came out in what year?
    1965

11. The Bond movie SPECTRE came out in what year?
    2015

12. The new version of Casino Royale came out in what year?
    2006

13. The TV version of Casino Royale was made in what year?
    1954

14. The Spy Who Loved Me came out in what year?
    1977

15. Moonraker came out in what year?
    1979

16. The Spy Who Loved Me came out in what year?
    1977

17. The Man with the Golden Gun came out in what year?
    1974

18. A View to a Kill came out in what year?
    1985

19. Which 2 Bond movies came out in 1983?
    Octopussy, Never Say Never Again

20. Tomorrow Never Dies came out in what year?
    1997

21. GoldenEye came out in what year?
    1995

22. Die Another Day came out in what year?
    2002

23. The World Is Not Enough came out in what year?
    1999

24. Licence to Kill came out in what year?
    1989

25. The Bond movie Quantum of Solace came out in what year?
    2008

26. On Die Another Day Jinx was the name of the Bond girl played by Halle Berry. Jinx told Bond she was born on what day?
    Friday the 13th

27. On the 1967 Casino Royale James Bond's nephew Jimmy Bond mentions his birthday is on what day?
    April Fool's Day

28. For Your Eyes Only came out in what year?
    1981

NUMBERS

1. On From Russia With Love and Thunderball Ernst Stavro Blofeld is what number in the S.P.E.C.T.R.E.organization?
   Number 1

2. On Thunderball Colonel Jacques Bouvar was what number in the S.P.E.C.T.R.E. organization?
   Number 6

3. On Goldfinger when a scientist defused Goldfinger's bomb in fort Knox what number did the bomb stop at?
   007

4. Desmond Llewelyn played "Q" on how many Bond movies?
   17

5. How many James Bond movies are called Casino Royale?
   3

6. At the beginning of From Russia with Love how long does it take for Red Grant to kill the intruder?
   1 minute and 52 seconds

7. At the beginning of Never Say Never Again how long did it take for Bond to wipe out an army of terrorists?
   1 minutes and 47 seconds

8. In On Her Majesty's Secret Service Draco bribes Bond to marry his daughter Tracy. How much does Draco bribe Bond with?
   1 million pounds in gold

9. At the beginning of A View to a Kill what Double O agent does Bond find dead in Siberia?
   Agent 003

10. What amount of money does Franz Sanchez bribe DEA agent Ed Killifer with to free him from the authorities on Licence to Kill?
    2 million dollars

11. On From Russia with Love what was the weight of the Lector Decoding machine?
    10 kilos

12. On You Only Live Twice Helga Brandt is what number in the S.P.E.C.T.R.E. organization?
    Number 11

13. On Never Say Never Again Largo is what number in the S.P.E.C.T.R.E. organization?
    Number 1

14. On Never Say Never Again Q Algernon tells Bond how many flavors of ice cream they have in the restaurant. What number of ice cream flavors did Algernon mention?
    28

15. Now that the Bond movies Skyfall and SPECTRE came out how many James Bond movies are there?
    27

16. What Double O agent was killed at the beginning of The Living Daylights?
    004

17. What Double O agent was killed on Octopussy?
    009

18. James Bond carries what Double O number?
    007

19. At the beginning of Never Say Never Again what does it say all over the screen when the movie and the theme song is starting?
    007

20. On Never Say Never Again Fatima Blush is what number in the S.P.E.C.T.R.E. organization?
    Number 12

21. Actor Robert Brown who played Admiral Hargreaves in The Spy Who Loved Me also played M in how many Bond movies?
    4

22. On GoldenEye when Alec Trevelyan was a Double O agent what Double O number did Trevelyan carry?
    006

23. On Thunderball Emilio Largo was what number in the crime organization S.P.E.C.T.R.E.?
    Number 2

24. On the James Bond movie SPECTRE the new car was assigned to what Double O agent?
    009

25. At the beginning of The Living Daylights when 3 Double O agents are on a training exercise which Double O agent gets captured by an S.A.S. soldier?
    Agent 002

DIRECTORS/PRODUCERS/SCREENWRITERS

1. Who was the director of the Bond movie Quantum of Solace?
   Marc Forster

2. The 1967 James Bond comedy Casino Royale was done by how many directors?
   5

3. Who were the 5 directors who did the 1967 James Bond comedy Casino Royale?
   John Huston, Kenneth Hughes, Val Guest, Robert Parrish, and Joe McGrath

4. Never Say Never Again was from the director of what Star Wars movie?
   The Empire Strikes Back

5. The 2006 Casino Royale was from the director of what other Bond movie?
   GoldenEye

6. Director Sam Mendes directed the two latest Bond movies Skyfall and SPECTRE. Sam Mendes also directed what two movies before Skyfall and SPECTRE?
   American Beauty and Road to Perdition

7. Which 3 Bond movies were directed by Terence Young?
   Dr. No, From Russia with Love and Thunderball

8. Which 4 Bond movies were directed by Guy Hamilton?
   Goldfinger, Diamonds Are Forever, Live and Let Die and The Man with the Golden Gun

9. Who was the director of Die Another Day?
   Lee Tamahori

10. Who was the screenwriter of You Only Live Twice?
    Roald Dahl

11. Who was the director of Tomorrow Never Dies?
    Roger Spottiswoode

12. Who was the director of The World Is Not Enough?
    Michael Apted

13. Who was the director of Never Say Never Again?
    Irvin Kershner

14. Who was the director of GoldenEye and the 2006 version of Casino Royale?
    Martin Campbell

15. Which 5 Bond movies were directed by John Glen?
    For Your Eyes Only, Octopussy, A View to a Kill, The Living Daylights, and Licence to Kill

16. Who was the director of the TV version of Casino Royale?
    William H. Brown

17. Who was the director of On Her Majesty's Secret Service?
    Peter Hunt

18. Marc Forster directed Daniel Craig's second James Bond movie Quantum of Solace. What 2018 movie did he also direct?
    Christopher Robin

19. Which 3 Bond movies were directed by Lewis Gilbert?
    You Only Live Twice, The Spy Who Loved Me, and Moonraker

WHICH NON-JAMES BOND MOVIE…

1. What Burt Reynolds comedy showed Roger Moore acting just like he did when he played James Bond?
   The Cannonball Run

2. Which Leslie Nielsen comedy was a spoof for James Bond and a few other movies?
   Spy Hard

3. Actor Richard Kiel played Jaws on The Spy Who Loved Me and Moonraker. Kiel had also appeared in which 1974 football movie starring Burt Reynolds?
   The Longest Yard

4. Before Richard Kiel played Jaws on The Spy Who Loved Me and Moonraker Kiel played an assassin with steel teeth on what 1976 comedy starring Gene Wilder and Richard Pryor?
   Silver Streak

5. Richard Kiel was a supporting actor on what Clint Eastwood western?
   Pale Rider

6. Richard Kiel played Jackie Chan's race partner on what Burt Reynolds comedy?
   Cannonball Run 2

7. Sean Connery played James Bond on Goldfinger in 1964. Connery also starred with Tippi Hedren on what Alfred Hitchcock movie in the same year?
   Marnie

8. What was the comedy spy movie series that was kind of a spoof of the James Bond series?
   Austin Powers

9. The helicopter chase scene on From Russia with Love was inspired by the crop duster chase scene on what Alfred Hitchcock movie?
   North by Northwest

10. The James Bond movie Moonraker came out in 1979. Which Monty Python movie came out in the same year?
    Monty Python's Life of Brian

11. Actor Peter Lorre played Le Chiffre on the 1954 TV play Casino Royale. 20 years before the TV version of Casino Royale Lorre played the villain on which Alfred Hitchcock classic that Hitchcock filmed two versions of?
    The Man Who Knew Too Much

12. On the 1967 Casino Royale George Raft had a cameo appearance where he flips a coin. Raft had a coin flipping role in what 1932 gangster movie?
    Scarface

13. Bond actor Roger Moore played Bond in the 1981 Bond movie For Your Eyes Only. Moore also co-starred in what Burt Reynolds comedy in the same year?
The Cannonball Run

14. On Austin Powers what was the name of the villain who was a spoof to Blofeld?
Dr. Evil

15. Which Rowan Atkinson comedy was kind of like a Mr. Bean spoof of James Bond?
Johnny English

16. Actor Art Malik played Kamran Shah on The Living Daylights. Malik also played the villian on what 1994 action movie starring Arnold Schwarzenegger, Jamie Lee Curtis, and Tom Arnold?
True Lies

17. Actor Clifton James played Sheriff J.W. Pepper on Live and Let Die and The Man with the Golden Gun. Clifton James also appeared on what 1976 comedy starring Gene Wilder and Richard Pryor?
Silver Streak

18. Actor Alec McCowen played Q Algernon in Never Say Never Again. McCowen had also played a Chief Inspector on what Alfred Hitchcock classic 11 years before Never Say Never Again?
Frenzy

19. Actor Barry Nelson played James Bond on the 1954 TV play Casino Royale. Barry Nelson had much later made an impressive appearance on which 1980 Horror movie based on a novel by Stephen King?
The Shining

20. Diamonds Are Forever came out in 1971. What family classic starring Gene Wilder came out in the same year?
Willy Wonka & the Chocolate Factory

21. The Spy Who Loved Me came out in 1977. What Burt Reynolds comedy came out in the same year?
Smokey and the Bandit

22. Diamonds Are Forever came out in 1971. Which 2 Clint Eastwood movies came out in the same year?
Dirty Harry and Play Misty for Me

23. Diamonds Are Forever came out in 1971. What action classic starring Gene Hackman came out in the same year?
The French Connection

24. No Bond movie came out in 1975 but what classic comedy came out in that year?
Monty Python and the Holy Grail

25. The Bond movie GoldenEye came out in 1995. What action movie starring Keanu Reeves, Dennis Hopper, and Sandra Bullock came out one year earlier?
Speed

26. The 1959 Alfred Hitchcock classic North by Northwest which is a lot like a James Bond movie came out how many years before James Bond 007 hit the big screen?
3 years

27. The Man with the Golden Gun came out in 1974. Which 2 Mel Brooks classics came out in the same year?
Young Frankenstein and Blazing Saddles

28. Diana Rigg who played Tracy in On Her Majesty's Secret Service also played which character on The Great Muppet Caper?
Lady Holiday

29. Actor Telly Savalas who played Blofeld in On Her Majesty's Secret Service is known for what TV role?
Kojak

30. Actor Mads Mikkelsen played Bond villain Le Chiffre on the 2006 remake of Casino Royale. Mikkelsen later played which character on the movie Rogue One: A Star Wars Story?
Galen Erso

31. Actor Daniel Craig played James Bond on 4 movies. Daniel Craig also starred on what 2011 remake of a 2009 movie based on the first of a book trilogy by Stieg Larsson?
The Girl with the Dragon Tattoo

32. Daniel Craig also teamed up with Harrison Ford on what 2011 movie that is a combination of western and Sci-Fi by the same director that did Iron Man?
Cowboys and Aliens

33. Actor Pierce Brosnan played James Bond on 4 movies. Brosnan also played Stuart Dunmeyer on what 1993 comedy classic starring Robin Williams and Sally Field?
Mrs. Doubtfire

34. Brosnan later played Sam, one of the three suitors on 2008's Mamma Mia The Movie. Brosnan later returned to the same role on what 2018 sequel?
Mamma Mia! Here We Go Again

35. Brosnan was also the lead actor on what 2014 movie that isn't a James Bond movie?
The November Man

36. Brosnan also played one of the bad guys on what 2017 action movie where Jackie Chan tries to find the bad guys who killed his daughter?
The Foreigner

37. Actor Sean Connery played James Bond on 7 movies. Sean Connery also played Indiana's father Professor Henry Jones on what 1989 Indiana Jones movie that is the third of the Indiana Jones trilogy?
    Indiana Jones and the Last Crusade

38. Actor Sean Connery played James Bond in 7 movies. Connery also played Edward Pierce on what 1978 action movie starring Sean Connery, Donald Sutherland, and Lesley-Anne Down?
    The Great Train Robbery

39. Actor Roger Moore played James Bond on 7 movies. Roger Moore also made a hilarious cameo as Peter Sellers' role Clouseau on what 1983 Pink Panther movie?
    Curse of the Pink Panther

40. Actor Sean Bean played Bond villain Alec Trevelyan on GoldenEye. Sean Bean also played terrorist Sean Miller on what 1992 action movie with Harrison Ford that was based on a novel by Tom Clancy?
    Patriot Games

41. Actor Sean Bean played Bond villain Alec trevelyan on the James Bond movie GoldenEye. Sean Bean also played what character on the Lord of the Rings trilogy?
    Boromir

42. Actress Famke Janssen played Xenia on GoldenEye. Janssen also played Liam Neeson's ex wife on which action movie trilogy?
    The Taken Trilogy

43. Actor Alan Cumming played computer programmer Boris Grishenko on GoldenEye. Alan Cumming also played which character on the Spy Kids movies?
    Fegan Floop

44. The first James Bond movie Dr. No came out in 1962. What Alfred Hitchcock movie came out two years earlier?
    Psycho

45. Actor Christopher Lee played Francisco Scaramanga on The Man with the Golden Gun. Christopher Lee also played which character on the Lord of the Rings trilogy?
    Saruman

46. Actor Christopher Lee played Francisco Scaramanga on The Man with the Golden Gun. Christopher Lee also played which character on two Star War prequels?
    Count Dooku

47. The comedy version of Casino Royale and the fifth Bond movie You Only Live Twice were released in 1967. What Disney movie came out in the same year?
    The Jungle Book

48. Actor David Niven played Sir James Bond on the comedy version of Casino Royale. Niven also played Sir Charles Litton the Phantom on what 3 Pink Panther movies?
    The Pink Panther, Trail of the Pink Panther, and Curse of the Pink Panther

49. Actor David Harbour played Gregg Beam on the James Bond movie Quantum of Solace. Harbour also played one of the bad guys on what action movie starring Denzel Washington?
    The Equalizer

MISCELLANEOUS TRIVIA

1. On the James Bond movie SPECTRE when Dr. Madeleine Swann asked James Bond what his position is James Bond says that his position doesn't look good on a form. Dr. Swan asked Bond what that is. What does James Bond tell her?
   James Bond tells her he kills people.

2. Mischka and Grischka perform what in Octopussy's circus?
   A daring knife throwing act while wearing blindfolds

3. On Never Say Never Again the Air Force performed what kind of test?
   They tried to perform a test with 2 dummy warheads.

4. What title did they almost give Licence to Kill?
   Licence Revoked

5. On Never Say Never Again when Blofeld talks about the abduction of 2 nuclear warheads the mouth of the silver metal skeleton head opens up. What comes out of its mouth before Blofeld starts talking?
   A video camera that records Blofeld talking

6. On the old Bond movies what cool thing does James Bond sometimes do when he steps into Miss Moneypenny's office?
   He takes off his hat, throws it at the hat rack and the hat rack catches the hat.

7. On The World Is Not Enough Q says 2 things he always tried to teach Bond. What were those 2 things?
   Never let them see you bleed, and always have an escape plan.

8. On For Your Eyes Only Timothy Havelock was what kind of worker?
   An archaeologist

9. What were the initials for On Her Majesty's Secret Service?
   OHMSS

10. What was the original title they almost gave A View to a Kill?
    From A View To A Kill

11. On the James Bond movie Skyfall how does James Bond try to protect M from getting killed by former agent Raoul Silva a.k.a. Tiago Rodriguez who is now a terrorist?
    James Bond takes M on his Aston Martin DB5 to his old childhood mansion called Skyfall and James Bond and M team up with Kincade as they set up traps and weapons in the Skyfall for when Silva and his men come to battle within Skyfall residence.

12. On Never Say Never Again when Bond and Largo played Domination against each other what color was Bond in the game and what color was Largo in the game?
    Bond was red and Largo was blue.

13. In On Her Majesty's Secret Service before the helicopter arrives at the Bleuchamp Institute Bunt tells Bond the place treats people with allergies. Bond said what kind of allergies? Bund said all of them. What 3 examples did she give for allergies?
    The hay fever, or the sickness caused by the oysters, or the inability to eat meat

14. In On Her Majesty's Secret Service when James Bond was in his office he looks at 3 souvenirs from 3 of his previous adventures. What were those 3 souvenirs?
    Honey Ryder's knife from Dr. No, Red Grant's wrist watch strangle wire from From Russia with Love, and James Bond's underwater breathing gadget from Thunderball

15. On Dr. No what was weird about Dr. No's hands?
    Dr. No had hands that look like black metal.

16. On The Spy Who Loved Me and Moonraker what was scary about Jaws the assassin?
    He had teeth that look like silver metal.

17. On the 1967 James Bond comedy Casino Royale Evelyn Tremble was an expert at what?
    Baccarat

18. On the 1967 James Bond comedy Casino Royale actor George Raft made a cameo appearance. What was his cameo appearance?
    He stood in the casino's bar and he flipped a coin.

19. Who played the voice of Blofeld on From Russia with Love and Thunderball when Anthony Dawson played Blofeld on those 2 Bond movies?
    Eric Pohlmann

20. What was unique about M from the old Bond movies to the new Bond movies?
    On the old Bond movies M is played by actors but on the new Bond movies M is played by an actress until Skyfall and SPECTRE.

21. On Dr. No what was Dr. No's nationality?
    German-Chinese

22. On the Bond movies how is James Bond known for how he sleeps at night?
    He sleeps with a gun under his pillow.

23. On Goldfinger there's a scene where James Bond finds Jill Masterson dead and her nude body covered in gold paint. Which scene from Quantum of Solace was similar to that scene?
    Bond's boss M shows James Bond that a woman he was involved with was killed and her body was covered in oil.

24. On Thunderball when James Bond and the Double O agents are in a meeting about the Thunderball mission a dossier was given to James Bond and the Double O agents. What are the 5 initials that appear on the cover of the dossier?
    OHMSS, which stands for On Her Majesty's Secret Service

25. On the 2006 Casino Royale what was the last line in the whole movie?
    "The name is Bond. James Bond."

26. On the 1967 Casino Royale what character was played by Kurt Kasznar?
    Smernov

27. On Thunderball what does S.P.E.C.T.R.E. do to conquer the world?
    Holding the world hostage with 2 hijacked atomic bombs

28. At the beginning of Never Say Never Again James Bond battles what kind of bad guys?
    Fanatical revolutionaries

29. In On Her Majesty's Secret Service when Bond is in his office what kind of picture does James Bond have in his office?
    A picture of the Queen

30. What was the name of the author who was the creator of James Bond?
    Ian Fleming

31. On Never Say Never Again Largo had a statuette. Who did the statuette belong to?
    Napoleon's Empress

32. On the 1967 Casino Royale what character was played by Charles Boyer?
    Le Grand

33. On Never Say Never Again when Bond is held prisoner in the dungeon Bond says to Largo "In this case where did you hide the bombs?" Largo tells Bond where Bomb #1 is but didn't tell Bond where Bomb #2 is. Where did Largo say Bomb #1 is?
    Under the President's feet in Washington D.C.

34. On The Man with the Golden Gun after the credits sequence when James Bond comes into M's office M shows Bond what they had received. What was it?
    A golden bullet that said 007 on it

35. On the Bond movies General Gogol is what kind of officer?
    KGB officer

36. At the beginning of From Russia with Love when Red Grant kills the intruder in S.P.E.C.T.R.E. island the intruder was what kind of intruder?
    A James Bond impersonator

37. On the 1967 Casino Royale what else does Le Chiffre do besides playing baccarat?
    Performs magic tricks

38. In On Her Majesty's Secret Service Bond asked Miss Moneypenny to have M accept his resignation from Her Majesty's Secret Service. Later what does Moneypenny have M give Bond instead of his resignation?
    Two weeks leave

39. At the beginning of Goldfinger who owned the heroin installation that is destroyed by Bond?
    Mr. Ramirez

40. On Never Say Never Again when Bond and Largo played Domination against each other what 5 countries did they fight for?
    France, Spain, Japan, the United States, and the rest of the World

41. On Octopussy what was Kamal Khan known as?
    An exiled Afghan prince

42. In On Her Majesty's Secret Service what is Blofeld known for?
    No earlobes

43. What was the name of the book that might have inspired Ian Fleming with the James Bond series?
    The book was called Birds of the West Indies by ornithologist names James Bond. So I think Ian Fleming named James Bond the secret agent after James Bond the ornithologist who wrote Birds of the West Indies

44. On the 1967 James Bond comedy Casino Royale how does Le Chiffre cheat at baccarat?
    By wearing x-ray eye glasses

45. On The Man with the Golden Gun what was the name of the thing Scaramanga needed for his villainous plot?
    Solex Agitator

46. On For Your Eyes Only what are the four things Milos Columbo likes to smuggle?
    Gold, diamonds, cigarettes, and pistachio nuts

47. On The Man with the Golden Gun what was abnormal about Scaramanga?
    Scaramanga had a third nipple.

48. On the 1967 Casino Royale Peter O'Toole appeared uncredited. Who did Peter O'Toole play?
    A recognised piper

49. On the James Bond movie Skyfall when Silva and his men destroy Bond's Aston Martin DB5 James Bond has a ticked off look on his face. What does James Bond do to get back at them?
    James Bond sets up the canisters to blow up his Skyfall mansion and then James Bond says to himself "I always hated this place."

50. On the 1967 Casino Royale when M and his men are in a car taking them to see Sir James Bond the road that leads to Bond's mansion was full of what kind of dangerous animals?
    Lions

51. On For Your Eyes Only what was the name of the talking parrot that belonged to the Havelock family?
    Max

52. On the 1967 Casino Royale during the casino fight scene bubbles go all around the casino. What kind of animal starts eating some of the bubbles?
    A monkey

53. On Live and Let Die what was the name of the crocodile that Tee Hee had accidentally lost his arm to?
    Old Albert

54. On the 1954 TV play Casino Royale Clarence Leiter thinks Zoltan looks like what kind of animal?
    A basset hound

55. On For Your Eyes Only Emile Locque is known as what in the Greek underworld?
    The Dove

56. Actor David Harbour played Gregg Beam on the James Bond movie Quantum of Solace. Harbour also played Chief Hopper on what 2016 science fiction TV series on Netflix?
    Stranger Things

"QUOTES"

1. On Dr. No when Sylvia says to Bond "I admire your luck Mr...." what does Bond say as he lights up a cigarette and James Bond music starts playing in the background?
   "Bond. James Bond."

2. On Tomorrow Never Dies what does Stamper say to Bond while trying to settle the score with Bond?
   "I owe you an unpleasant death Mr. Bond."

3. On Moonraker when Bond throws Chang out the window what does Bond say after Chang fell through a piano?
   "Play it again Sam."

4. On You Only Live Twice after Bond faked his assassination while Bond is in the submarine he enters Miss Moneypenny's office. Miss Moneypenny says to Bond, "You're late as usual. Even from your own funeral." What does Bond say?
   "Well we corpses have absolutely no sense of time."

5. On Goldfinger what does Bond say after he electrocutes Capungo?
   "Shocking. Positively shocking."

6. On From Russia with Love after Rosa Klebb dies Tatiana Romanova says, "Horrible woman." What does Bond say?
   "She's had her kicks."

7. On Moonraker what does Bond say to Drax before Drax gets sucked out into space?
   "Take a giant step for mankind."

8. On GoldenEye when Alec Trevelyan almost fell to his death James Bond catches Trevelyan's foot. Trevelyan said, "For England James?" What does Bond say before he let go of Trevelyan's foot?
   "No. For me."

9. On The World Is Not Enough when Renard says to Bond, "You can't kill me. I'm already dead" what does Bond say?
   "Not dead enough for me."

10. On For Your Eyes Only what does Bond say to Columbo and his men after Emile Leopold Locque fell to his death in his car?
    "He had no head for heights."

11. On Tomorrow Never Dies when Dr. Kaufman says to Bond "Wait. I'm just a professional doing a job" what does Bond say before he shoots Dr. Kaufman in the head?
    "Me too."

12. On Licence to Kill when Bond sees the underground water full of sharks what does Bond say to Killifer?
"Is this where you stuck your old buddy Felix?"

13. On Licence to Kill when Killifer almost fell into the water full of sharks he grabs a rope that saves him from falling. Killifer says to Bond, "There's 2 million in the briefcase. We can split the money." What does Bond say before he throws the briefcase on Killifer?
"You want it. You keep it Old Buddy!"

14. After Bond threw the briefcase on Killifer, Killifer accidentally let go of the rope, the briefcase opened as Killifer fell into the sharks. Bond and Sharkey watched Killifer get killed by the sharks while the 2 million dollars were all over the water and the dollars were all wet and destroyed. What does Sharkey say?
"What a terrible waste. Of money."

15. On GoldenEye when Alec Trevelyan says to Bond, "Why can't you just be a good boy and die?" what does Bond say?
"You first."

16. On GoldenEye when Bond knocks Xenia unconscious what does he say to her?
"Sweet dreams."

17. On The Man with the Golden Gun when Bond says to Scaramanga "six bullets to your one?" what does Scaramanga say?
"I only need one."

18. On For Your Eyes Only when Kristatos and his men were getting ready to feed Bond and Melina to the sharks what does Kristatos say to his men?
"Leave the legs free. They'll make appetizing bait."

19. On The Spy Who Loved Me what does Bond say after Sandor fell to his death?
"What a helpful chap."

20. On Live and Let Die what does Quarrel Jr. say to Bond before Bond goes to save Miss Solitaire from voodoo cultists and before Quarrel Jr. blows up Dr. Kananga's poppy fields?
"My regards to Baron Samedi man. Right between the eyes."

21. In On Her Majesty's Secret Service when Blofeld says to Bond, "So first a little therapy to soothe your restless nature," Bond sees Campbell's corpse hanging upside down outside the window. What does Blofeld say?
"Poor fellow. He was restless too."

22. On The World Is Not Enough when Renard had Davidov using Dr. Arkov's identity to get on a plane taking him to a nuclear site where Renard and his men were up to no good, Bond kills Davidov before he can catch that plane. Bond dumps the corpse into the trash. Soon after that a man from the plane says to Bond, "Where's Davidov? I was told to expect him." What does Bond say with a smile?
"He was buried with work."

23. On Tomorrow Never Dies when Bond said "accidents do happen" what does Q say?
"They frequently do with you."

24. On From Russia with Love when it showed a billboard of Anita Ekberg on a building Krilencu tries to climb out of Anita's mouth. What does Bond say after Krilencu is shot and killed?
"She should've kept her mouth shut."

25. On Thunderball what does Bond say after he killed Vargas in self defense?
"I think he got the point."

26. On Live and Let Die what does Bond say after Dr. Kananga blows up from the shark gun?
"He always did have an inflated opinion about himself."

27. On The Spy Who Loved Me when Bond finds Fekkesh dead Anya says, "Where's Fekkesh?" What did Bond say?
"With the Pharaohs."

28. On The Spy Who Loved Me what does Bond say after the bad guy on a motorcycle gets covered in feathers and falls to his death?
"All those feathers and he still can't fly."

29. On Licence to Kill when Bond and Pam found that Heller was killed with a forklift blade what does Bond say about Heller?
"He must've come to a dead end."

30. On From Russia with Love after Bond kills Red Grant what does Bond say to the corpse?
"You won't be needing this anymore old man."

31. On Moonraker when Corinne says "Welcome to California Mr. Bond" what does Bond say?
"I like it already."

32. In On Her Majesty's Secret Service when Bond says "Moneypenny what would I do without you?" what does Miss Moneypenny say?
"My only problem is that you'd never do anything with me."

33. On GoldenEye what does Xenia Onatopp say to James Bond before she tries to suffocate him with her thighs?
"This time Mr. Bond the pleasure will be all mine."

34. On Dr. No what does Miss Moneypenny say to James Bond about flirting?
"Flattery will get you nowhere but don't stop trying."

35. On The Man with the Golden Gun when James Bond says "Moneypenny you are better than a computer" what does Miss Moneypenny say?
"In all sorts of ways."

36. In On Her Majesty's Secret Service when Tracy shows up in Bond's hotel room holding Bond's gun Bond says "You're full of surprises Contessa" what does Tracy say?
"So are you Mr. Bond. Do you always arm yourself for a rendezvous?"

37. In On Her Majesty's Secret Service when Miss Moneypenny says to James Bond "Where have you been?" what does James Bond say?
"Much too far from you darling."

38. In On Her Majesty's Secret Service when Tracy says to Draco, "Mr Bond and I have already met" what does Bond say?
"But each time is a renewed pleasure."

39. On Never Say Never Again when Bond says to Fatima Blush "you appear tense," what does Fatima Blush say?
"You affect me James."

40. In On Her Majesty's Secret Service what does Bond say to Tracy as she helps him escape from Bunt and Blofeld's thugs?
"Thank you Tracy. You've got sharp eyes and beautiful...earlobes."

41. On Moonraker when Holly kisses Bond Bond says "What was that for?" Holly says "For saving my life." What does Bond say?
"Remind me to do it more often."

42. At the end of On Her Majesty's Secret Service what memorable quote does Bond say to his wife Tracy before she gets shot and killed?
"We have all the time in the world."

43. On The Spy Who Loved Me when Bond tells Felicca that he already ate when Felicca tries to be romantic to him what does Bond say before they kiss?
"But I seem to have missed dessert."

44. At the beginning of On Her Majesty's Secret Service what does James Bond say after Tracy leaves the beach?
"This never happened to the other fellow."

45. On The Man with the Golden Gun what does James Bond say when Andrea Anders shows up in Bond's hotel room?
"Mrs. Anders. I didn't recognize you with your clothes on."

46. On From Russia with Love when Tatiana Romanova says to Bond "But I think my mouth is too big" what does Bond say before they kiss?
"No it's the right size. For me that is."

47. The World Is Not Enough when Q introduces Bond to the fellow Q was grooming as his replacement, what does Bond say to Q?
"You're Q. Doesn't that make him R?"

48. In On Her Majesty's Secret Service what does Blofeld say to one of his thugs while James Bond was skiing out of Piz Gloria?
"We'll head him off at the precipice."

49. On Never Say Never Again when Lippe tries to kill Bond at Shrublands Health Spa Bond and Lippe go all over the place fighting each other and do terrible damage to the Clinic. After Lippe dies it goes to the next scene. On the next scene what does M say to Bond?
"I send you to a health farm to get yourself in shape. Instead you demolish it. I've had to notify the local police, throw out the special branch, get the Minister to muzzle the press, and allocate a sizeable chunk of my meager budget to renovating the establishment."

50. On Thunderball what does Bond say to Felix Leiter when Felix and his men rescued Bond in a plane?
"Get your radio men on to Orlando Beach. Warn them the target is Miami."

51. On The Man with the Golden Gun when Andrea Anders says to Bond "Why should you trust me?" what does Bond say?
"I don't. But neither will Mr. Scaramanga trust you if he hears about our little conversation. Why who knows? He might use one of those little golden bullets on you. And that would be a pity because they're very expensive."

52. On Octopussy when Magda says to James Bond, "He suggests a trade. The egg for your life" what does James Bond say?
"I'd hear the price of eggs is going up but isn't that a little high?"

53. In On Her Majesty's Secret Service when Draco says to Bond "My apologies for how you were brought here. Please sit down. I wasn't sure you'd accept a formal invitation" what does Bond say?
"There's always something formal about the point of a pistol."

54. On Licence to Kill what does M say to Bond after Bond refuses to obey M's orders?
"We're not a country club 007. Effective immediately your licence to kill is revoked."

55. On From Russia with Love what does Bond say to Red Grant soon before Grant slaps Bond in the face?
"Tell me, which lunatic asylum did they get you out of?"

56. On Never Say Never Again when Bond tries to sneak past the man in charge of the guest list, the man tries to stop Bond, Bond punches the man in the stomach and some guests come in while Bond was walking the man into a room. The man was in pain and had his hand on his stomach. What does Bond say to the guests who were walking in?
"You shouldn't have the fish."

57. On Octopussy what did Kamal Khan say to James Bond when Bond was staying with Octopussy?
"You have a nasty habit of surviving."

58. On For Your Eyes Only what Chineses proverb does Bond say to Melina about the vendetta she seeks?
"Before setting out on revenge, you first dig 2 graves."

59. On The World Is Not Enough when Electra King says to Bond "I could've given you the world" what does Bond say?
"The World Is Not Enough."

60. On Moonraker when Corinne Dufour takes Bond to start his tour at a building of Drax's what does Drax say to Chang?
"Look after Mr. Bond. See that some harm comes to him."

61. On The Man with the Golden Gun when Scaramanga says to Bond "You get as much fulfillment out of killing as I do so why don't you admit it?" what does Bond say?
"I admit killing you would be a pleasure."

62. On Never Say Never Again after Bond beat Largo at his own game Domination Largo says to Bond "Do you lose as gracefully as you win?" what does Bond say?
"I don't know. I've never lost."

63. On Live and Let Die what does the cab driver say after Bond pays him?
"Sure hope you make friends easy. Right on Brother."

64. On The Spy Who Loved Me when Bond was in Stromberg's office that was full of aquariums Bond says to Stromberg "Do you miss the outside world?" What does Stomberg say?
"For me, this is all the world. There is beauty...there is ugliness...and there is death."

65. On The World Is Not Enough when Mr. Lachaise says to Bond "I'm giving you the chance to walk out with the money" what does Bond say?
"And I'm giving you the chance to walk out with your life."

66. On Never Say Never Again when Fatima Blush says to Bond "How wreckless of me. I got you all wet" what does Bond say?
"Yes but my martini is still dry."

67. On Live and Let Die when Dr. Kananga said "What shall we drink to Mr. Bond?" what does James Bond say?
"How about an earthquake?"

68. On The Man with the Golden Gun when Bond was with Lazar what did Lazar say about the bullet?
"It's not the bullet that kills. It's the finger that pulls the trigger."

69. In On Her Majesty's Secret Service when Bond and Fraulein Irma Bunt are in the helicopter what does Fraulein Bunt say when the helicopter takes off?
"Now up into ze Alps."

70. On the 1967 Casino Royale what does Jimmy Bond say when a firing squad gets ready to shoot him?

"You do know this means an angry letter to the Times."

We hope you enjoyed *The Game's Trivia.... James Bond Trivia*.

You can find all of our books, including another book featuring Chad, *Treasures of Darkness: Unwrapping the Gift of Autism*, at www.brendenbooks.com.

Chad & Sally Brenden

Printed in Great Britain
by Amazon

15809429R00050